Patients' Guide to

Cervical Cancer

Uni
Ca
Gy

Breast
s and
ursing

World Headquarters
Jones and Bartlett Publishers
40 Tall Pine Drive
Sudbury, MA 01776
978-443-5000
info@jbpub.com
www.jbpub.com

Jones and Bartlett Publishers
Canada
6339 Ormindale Way
Mississauga, Ontario L5V 1J2
Canada

Jones and Bartlett Publishers
International
Barb House, Barb Mews
London W6 7PA
United Kingdom

Jones and Bartlett's books and products are available through most bookstores and online booksellers. To contact Jones and Bartlett Publishers directly, call 800-832-0034, fax 978-443-8000, or visit our website at www.jbpub.com.

Substantial discounts on bulk quantities of Jones and Bartlett's publications are available to corporations, professional associations, and other qualified organizations. For details and specific discount information, contact the special sales department at Jones and Bartlett via the above contact information or send an email to specialsales@jbpub.com.

The author, editors, and publisher have made every effort to provide accurate information. However, they are not responsible for errors, omissions, or for any outcomes related to the use of the contents of this book and take no responsibility for the use of the products and procedures described. Treatments and side effects described in this book may not be applicable to all people; likewise, some people may require a dose or experience a side effect that is not described herein. Drugs and medical devices are discussed that may have limited availability controlled by the Food and Drug Administration (FDA) for use only in a research study or clinical trial. Research, clinical practice, and government regulations often change the accepted standard in this field. When consideration is being given to use of any drug in the clinical setting, the healthcare provider or reader is responsible for determining FDA status of the drug, reading the package insert, and reviewing prescribing information for the most up-to-date recommendations on dose, precautions, and contraindications, and determining the appropriate usage for the product. This is especially important in the case of drugs that are new or seldom used.

Production Credits
Executive Publisher: Christopher Davis
Editorial Assistant: Sara Cameron
Associate Production Editor: Lisa Cerrone
Senior Marketing Manager: Barb Bartoszek
V.P., Manufacturing and Inventory Control: Therese Connell
Composition: Appingo Publishing Services
Cover Design: Kristin E. Parker
Cover Image: © ImageZoo/age fotostock
Printing and Binding: Malloy, Inc.
Cover Printing: Malloy, Inc.

Library of Congress Cataloging-in-Publication Data

McCormick, Colleen C.
   Johns Hopkins medicine patients' guide to cervical cancer / Colleen C. McCormick, Robert L. Giuntoli ; series editors, Lillie D. Shockney, Gary R. Shapiro.
      p. cm. — (Johns Hopkins patients' guide series)
   Includes index.
   ISBN 978-0-7637-7427-1 (pbk.)
   1. Cervix uteri—Cancer—Popular works. I. Giuntoli, Robert L. II. Title. III. Title: Patients' guide to cervical cancer.
   RC280.U8G48 2011
   616.99'466—dc22

                                                                              2009048265

6048

Printed in the United States of America

14 13 12 11 10   10 9 8 7 6 5 4 3 2 1

DEDICATION

This book is dedicated to all my patients, especially those with cervical cancer. I continued to be humbled by the strength demonstrated by these women and their families. I hope these chapters serve as a meaningful resource to help guide you in your journey toward restored health.

To my family—Svetlana, Anastasia, and Alexandra—for your invaluable love and support that have made this book possible.

Robert L. Giuntoli, II

Contents

PREFACE

Receiving a diagnosis of cervical cancer is over-whelming. Trying to determine your next steps following the diagnosis can be equally paralyzing. Rather than entering an environment that is totally foreign to you, consider learning some information in advance.

With more than 11,270 women diagnosed with cervical cancer in the United States in 2009, you are certainly not alone. Many have come before you, and still more will come after you. Empowering yourself with information is key to making informed decisions, participating in treatment choices presented to you by your oncology team, and gaining confidence that you are on the right track.

This book is part of a series of Johns Hopkins cancer patient guides designed to educate newly diagnosed patients about their cancer diagnosis and the treatment that may lie ahead. The information provided will guide patients and their support teams of family and friends from the time cancer is confirmed to the time treatment is completed.

Don't feel the need to read the entire book at once. It is intended for you to read it at your leisure and when you feel ready for additional information. Resource information, including access to Johns Hopkins oncology specialists, is also contained within these pages.

Until there is a cure, the team of the Kelly Gynecologic Oncology Service will continue to support patients who hear the words "you have cervical cancer."

Colleen C. McCormick, MD

Robert L. Giuntoli, II, MD

INTRODUCTION

HOW TO USE THIS BOOK TO YOUR BENEFIT

You will receive a great deal of information from your healthcare team. You will also probably seek out some information on the Internet or in bookstores. No doubt friends and family members, meaning well, will offer you advice on what to do and when to do it, and will try to steer you in certain directions. Relax. Yes, you have heard words you wish you had never heard said about you, that you have cervical cancer. Despite that, you have time to make good decisions and to empower yourself with accurate information so that you can participate in the decision making about your care and treatment.

This book is designed to be a how-to guide that will take you through the maze of treatment options and sometimes complicated schedules, and will help you to put together a plan of action so that you become a cervical cancer survivor. In the United States, seventy-one percent of women diagnosed today will be survivors of this disease. The statistics are even better for early-stage disease, of which ninety-two percent will be cured. Your goal is to join that majority.

The book is broken down into chapters and includes an index as well as credible resources listed for your further review and education. By empowering yourself with understandable information, we hope you will be comfortable participating in the decision making about your treatment.

Cervical cancers are serious and need to be treated expediently, but you need to understand and be comfortable with your physician's recommendations. With few exceptions, you have time to plan things well and confidently.

Let's begin now with understanding what has happened and what the steps are to get you well again.

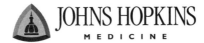

First Steps—
I've Been Diagnosed
with Cervical Cancer

Women often have one of two reactions to being told they have cervical cancer. If they have been having Pap smears, they may feel confused: "But I had a normal Pap smear last time! How did this happen?" And if they haven't had a Pap smear in a while, they may feel guilty: "I should have seen the doctor sooner." Either way, the diagnosis can be devastating. Cervical cancer may be difficult for women to discuss because it involves the cervix (the opening of the womb), which is not a part of the body women usually talk about. Also cervical cancer is caused by a sexually transmitted virus, and women might feel embarrassed. Let's deal with these issues first.

ANATOMY

The anatomy of the female pelvis is not necessarily a familiar area. Many important parts are located in the pelvis and it may be helpful to review the anatomy before moving forward.

The reproductive organs include the uterus (the womb), the cervix, the fallopian tubes, and the ovaries. The uterus sits in the middle of the pelvis and the fallopian tubes and ovaries are located to the right and the left. The cervix is the opening to the uterus and is the part that dilates when a woman goes into labor. The cervix is divided into two parts. The ectocervix is the outside portion of the cervix and is lined by squamous cells. The endocervix is the inside portion of the cervix. It is the tunnel that leads to the inside of the uterus and is lined by glandular cells. The labia (lips) are the part of the female genitalia that you see on the outside and are sometimes referred to as the vulva or genitalia. The vagina (birth canal) connects the cervix to the vulva, and as the name implies, this is the tunnel that babies travel through when they are born (unless a cesarean section is performed). The rectum and sigmoid colon (where bowel movement is stored) are located behind the uterus and cervix. The bladder (where urine is stored) is located in front of the uterus and cervix. **Figure 1-1** has been included for easy reference.

When you go to the gynecologist's office for a routine exam, the doctor will evaluate all these organs. The gynecologist first looks at the outside to make sure there are no abnormal areas. He or she then inserts an instrument called a speculum to look at the cervix and vagina. The bimanual exam is the part of the exam where the doctor uses his or her hands to feel for abnormalities of the uterus, cervix, tubes, and ovaries. A rectal exam is often performed to better evaluate the pelvis.

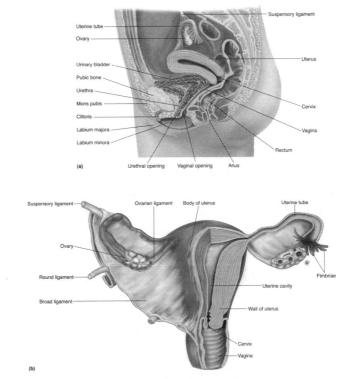

Figure 1-1   Anatomy of the female reproductive system.

If there is a suspicion of cervical cancer or if cervical cancer has been diagnosed, surgery may be recommended. These procedures will be discussed in detail in later chapters, but a short introduction will be helpful as we proceed forward. Knowledge of the anatomy is essential for an understanding of the surgery. A cold knife cone and a loop electrosurgical excisional procedure (LEEP) involve removal of part of the cervix. They are often performed to make a diagnosis, but can sometimes be sufficient to cure the disease. A trachelectomy refers to removal of the cervix without removal of the uterus. This procedure preserves fertility. A total hysterectomy involves removal of the uterus and cervix. The type of hysterectomy just refers to how the uterus is removed. If the tubes and ovaries are removed, this is referred to as a salpingo-oophorectomy, and can involve both the right and left or just one side.

WHAT CAUSES CERVICAL CANCER?

Cervical cancer and the precancerous entity dysplasia are caused by a virus called human papillomavirus (called HPV for short). There are many different types of HPV, some of which cause warts and some of which can cause cervical dysplasia and cancer.

HPV is sexually transmitted, and may be likened to a sexually transmitted common cold. Of women who are sexually active, 85% will be infected with HPV within the first 3 years of having sex. So pretty much everyone gets HPV. Usually the virus infects and irritates the cells on the cervix. Most of the time our bodies fight off the infection, and it goes away without causing any problems. Sometimes, either because our immune system isn't working as well as it should or for reasons we still don't understand, our body doesn't fight off the virus. Smoking can also interfere with your immune system's ability to remove the virus. If your body doesn't get rid of the HPV infection, you can develop cervical dysplasia, which, if left untreated for years, can become a cervical cancer.

HOW DO WE PREVENT CERVICAL CANCER?

Papanicolaou (Pap) smears are designed to find evidence of persistent HPV infection (an infection that won't go away) on your cervix. Usually, Pap smears allow doctors to find precancers (cervical dysplasia) before they develop into cancer. If cell changes are noted early, doctors often simply watch to make sure your cervix is doing its job of fighting off the infection. If these changes are more advanced, doctors often intervene to eliminate the abnormal cells.

Unfortunately, Pap smears are not perfect; they only find changes, if there are any, about 60% of the time. That's why we have to do Pap smears so often. Since it usually takes at least 5–10 years for irritation from an HPV infection to cause cancer, this system works pretty well. However, Pap smears sometimes don't pick up the changes until after cancer has already developed. This delayed detection happens most often when the HPV infection affects the cervical canal rather than the outside of the cervix. Even in these situations, the cancer is still identified at an early stage.

If you haven't had a Pap smear in a while, you may be feeling guilty. There are lots of reasons why women don't get Pap smears, and beating yourself up over it will take your energy away from fighting your cancer.

Once again, it's important to note that smoking increases the risk of developing cervical cancer and dysplasia and worsens the outcome for women who have developed cervical cancer. Therefore, smoking cessation is a great idea both for women who are at risk for cervical cancer or dysplasia and for women who have already developed cervical disease. As a cancer patient or survivor, sharing your thoughts with a friend or family member may be enough to stop someone from smoking and can make a tremendous difference in someone's health.

WHAT ABOUT VACCINES?

Vaccines are medicines that result in immunity against infections. They teach your immune system how to fight a particular virus or bacteria. Vaccines can be either pro-phylactic or therapeutic. A prophylactic vaccine prevents an infection from occurring. It doesn't work in someone who has already been infected. A therapeutic vaccine treats a patient after she has already been infected with the disease.

A prophylactic vaccine that prevents genital warts and the majority of cervical cancers is currently available. The vaccine prevents infection by HPV 6 and 11, which cause warts, and HPV 16 and 18, which cause two-thirds of cervical cancers. Unfortunately, the vaccine does not work in women who have already been infected. The vaccine is recommended in girls ages 11–12, with catch-up vac-cination recommended for females ages 13–26. Even if a patient is vaccinated, she still needs to get Pap smears as recommended. Although women with dysplasia have been infected with at least one HPV type, it is extremely unlikely for anyone to be infected with all four HPV types covered by the vaccine. Therefore, patients with dysplasia are still eligible for the vaccine. In these cases, the vaccine will not make the dysplasia go away, but can prevent infection by other HPV types. The vaccine is not recommended for patients with cervical cancer.

Clinical trials will continue to investigate therapeutic vac-cines for HPV. However, these trials are in their early stages and there are no commercially available therapeutic HPV vaccines. Unfortunately, current vaccines are not helpful for women already diagnosed with cervical cancer.

As a cervical cancer patient or survivor, you are uniquely po-sitioned to educate your friends and family about the HPV vaccine. You may be the difference between someone get-ting or not getting the vaccine. Although the vaccine won't prevent your cervical cancer, you could play a vital role in preventing someone else from getting cervical cancer.

OK, so now that we've covered some basics, let's talk about getting your treatment started.

SELECTING AN ONCOLOGIST/MEDICAL CENTER

Women with cervical cancer should be treated by a gynecologic oncologist. Gynecologic oncologists are doctors who have received specialty training to operate and give chemotherapy for cancers that only women can develop (such as cervical, ovarian, and uterine cancers). Gynecologic oncologists are certified by the American Board of Obstetrics and Gynecology. You should make sure that your physician is either board certified or board eligible. Studies have shown that women who contract these types of cancers and are treated by gynecologic oncologists typically receive better care, have a lower recurrence rate, and have a higher survival rate. The easiest way to find out if your doctor is board certified is to ask her or him directly.

After the diagnosis of cervical cancer has been made, your gynecologist will usually give a referral to a gynecologic oncologist. This is a good first step. As with any significant health care decision, a second opinion can be appropriate. There are many sources for a second opinion. A friend or family member may have required treatment by a gynecologic oncologist. The Internet can also be a good resource. Patients can search for gynecologic oncologists in their area on Web sites such as the Women's Cancer Network (http://www.wcn.org/).

Gynecologic oncologists can practice in an academic center or in a community hospital. Both systems provide excellent

7

care, but have several differences. Some patients prefer academic centers, while others prefer community hospitals. Additionally, some medical centers are hybrids of both systems.

Gynecologic oncologists are experts who help you survive and cope with what is happening to you. Always make sure your doctor is someone you feel comfortable with and that he or she is willing to explain the procedures you are about to have. Remember, your doctor is there for you!

In addition to choosing your physician, you have a choice of facilities in which to receive care. There are certain features that are considered valuable characteristics in a cancer center. Does the facility provide easy access with timely appointments? Is the facility committed to having the patient as an active participant in treatment planning? Are there resources available for patient and family education? Is there a multidisciplinary conference to review patient treatment recommendations? Can all your treatment (surgery, chemotherapy, and radiation) be performed within the cancer center?

LEARNING MORE ABOUT YOUR DISEASE BEFORE THE FIRST VISIT

Cervical precancers (dysplasia) have not yet invaded the cervix and can *all* be cured with a procedure to remove a piece of your cervix (usually a LEEP or a cone, discussed in Chapter 3). Even women with cervical cancers that are detected early have a good chance of long-term survival. In fact, more than 70% of women with cervical cancer will survive for 5 years or longer and are considered cured.

As we learn more about the behavior of cervical cancers and dysplasias, we have become more comfortable with less radical treatment of these diseases. One important development is that we can obtain the same cure rates with fewer side effects. In most cases, long-term cure can be achieved with little impact in long-term quality of life. In fact in most cases of cervical dysplasia and some cases of early stage cervical cancer, treatment can be obtained while still maintaining your ability to become pregnant and deliver a baby. These issues will be discussed in more detail in subsequent chapters.

The first step in treatment is to determine the stage of disease. Your gynecologic oncologist will "stage you" to determine how advanced your cancer is and the related procedures that may or may not be required at that time.

GATHERING RECORDS: BIOPSY, LABS, RADIOLOGY REPORTS

It is a good idea for you to start a binder for keeping copies of all important documents about your cancer care. Request copies of your medical records, including, but not limited to, pathology reports, radiology reports, and operative notes. Keep copies of everything as you continue treatment so you have information about your care.

These records are necessary for your gynecologic oncologist to figure out the best treatment plan for you. Likely, your cancer or dysplasia was diagnosed on a biopsy. You may have had a colposcopy (a procedure in which the doctor looks at your cervix with a magnifying glass). Your gynecologic oncologist can best start planning your treatment if he or she has a copy of the colposcopy findings, the operative notes from any procedures you had (LEEP or cone), pathology reports, and any radiology reports. Your gynecologic oncologist will also want to see the actual films/images from any CAT (computerized axial tomography) scans you had and will want to have the pathologists at his or her medical center review the actual pathology slides from any biopsies or procedures you have had.

You might think, "Why do I need to get these things if my doctors have the reports?" An accredited cancer center usually reviews the relevant images and the pathology slides from other institutions in order to verify their accuracy. There are situations in which review by a specialist in cervical pathology reveals an error was made and that instead of invasive cervical cancer, the patient has non-invasive disease. Of course, the opposite situation is also possible, and the pathologist may change the diagnosis from "benign" or noninvasive to invasive cervical cancer. Accuracy is key for pathology. Your treatment plan at every step is based on this information being correct.

CANCER STAGING

The term "stage" is a fancy way of saying how advanced your cancer is. If you have cervical dysplasia, this precancerous process is usually not staged, though in some cases as explained below, it may be called "stage 0." If you have a cervical cancer, the recommended treatment depends a lot on what stage your cancer is, so let's jump-start your knowledge base before your doctor's visit.

The stage of a cervical cancer is determined clinically, meaning that your gynecologic oncologist uses the findings from a physical examination and several basic tests to determine your stage. Once you are diagnosed with a stage, you will always have that stage—even if your cancer goes away or comes back. To determine your stage, your doctor will probably do an "exam under anesthesia," a cystoscopy, and a sigmoidoscopy. Although this series of tests is done in the operating room, it is a "same-day procedure," and you will be able to go home when it is done. The anesthesia is given to relax you so the doctor can do a thorough pelvic exam and determine the exact size of your cervical cancer. During the cystoscopy, the doctor will look in your bladder with a small camera. During the sigmoidoscopy, the doctor will make sure the cancer has not spread to the rectal area. Although not part of official staging, doctors often order a CAT scan to determine if the cancer has spread beyond the cervix.

The stage of your cancer will determine what treatment you will receive and is also tied to survival estimates. However, you are not a statistic; you are a person, and people fall on both sides of these estimates.

Dysplasia is a precancer of the cervix. Dysplasias involve just the lining of the cervix. Unlike cancers, dysplasias do not invade the cervix. Dysplasias are divided into mild, moderate, and severe. The grading is based on the extent to which the lining of the cervix is involved. Mild dysplasia only involves one-third of the lining. Severe dysplasia involves over two-thirds of the lining. Carcinoma in situ occurs when dysplasia involves the entire thickness of the lining. It is the last step before cancer, but it is *not* yet cancer because it has not invaded the cervix. Carcinoma in situ is sometimes referred to as stage 0 cervical cancer. Basically, carcinoma in situ means the cervical cells have become *almost* cancer. As discussed in Chapter 3, surgery (a LEEP or cone) will likely be recommended to remove the precancer and to make sure there is no area that has already become cancerous.

Stage I cancer has not spread beyond the cervix. It is further subclassified as stage IA1, IA2, IB1, and IB2, which are explained in more detail in Chapter 3. In stage IA cancers, the disease is still so small that it can only be detected by a microscope. Stage IB cancer is large enough that a doctor can see the cancer, but it still involves only the cervix and has not spread to the vagina or elsewhere. For an anatomic overview and a diagram of the female reproductive organs, please see the anatomy section of this chapter and **Figure 1-1**.

Stage II cancer has spread to involve the top part of the vagina or the ligaments that hold the cervix in place.

Stage III cancer has spread down to the lower part of the vagina or all the way to the sidewall (or bones) of the pelvis.

Stage IV cancer (known as metastatic cancer) involves the bladder or rectum, or it has spread to more distant places like the lung, liver, or bone.

In general, stage I cervical cancer is treated with surgery or with radiation and chemotherapy, and later stage cancer is treated with radiation and chemotherapy.

CERVICAL CANCER AND FERTILITY

Cervical cancer can develop in women while they are still young and have not begun or finished having children. Because the cervix is part of the uterus, treatment of cervical cancer can mean that the uterus will have to be removed or that it will be exposed to radiation. Some early cervical cancers can be treated with a procedure (known as a trachelectomy) that removes the cervix but leaves the uterus in place. However, this approach is not always a possibility. It's important to have a discussion with your gynecologic oncologist about your desires for future childbearing before you begin treatment. If necessary, a referral can be made to a specialist in reproductive endocrinology and infertility.

These physicians specialize in taking care of women with infertility or special needs that may make getting pregnant more challenging.

Obviously, the best way to preserve your fertility is to avoid radiation and to preserve your uterus, tubes, and ovaries, and as much of your cervix as possible. Unfortunately, with cervical cancer this often is not a realistic possibility. However, even if reproductive organs need to be removed for treatment of your cervical cancer, options for future fertility remain. If your uterus needs to be removed but your ovarian function has been preserved, in vitro fertilization could be used to create a pregnancy, which can be carried by a surrogate (somebody willing to be pregnant for you). Sometimes your eggs, or even whole ovaries, can be harvested prior to treatment and frozen for use at a later date. However, this technique is still in its infancy and is considered experimental. For some women adoption may often prove to be the best option. Even if you are unsure of your plans to have children, losing the possibility may be difficult, and counseling or support groups can be helpful in dealing with this loss. As mentioned above, the discussion about future fertility often begins with your gynecologic oncologist. The more extensive your treatment recommendations become, the more likely a referral to an infertility specialist will be reasonable. A referral can be obtained through your gynecologic oncologist. In addition, Web sites are available to find physicians in your area. The American Society of Reproductive Medicine provides a "Find a Doctor" link at their Web site: http://www.asrm.org/. If you would like children and decide to proceed with adoption, many reputable organizations and websites are available for assistance.

Finally, considering fertility and trying to maximize your options for the future is a smart approach. However, you also need to keep sight of the issue at hand. The first order of business is to fully evaluate and appropriately treat the cervical cancer. As long as the treatment plan takes into consideration your desires to have children in the future, you can revisit the issue of fertility once the dust has settled.

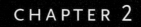

CHAPTER 2

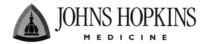

My Team—Meeting Your Treatment Team

PLAYERS

Your oncology team begins with your diagnosis and consists of many members from different areas. Each person plays a key role that is instrumental in helping you deal with the many facets of cervical cancer care.

CERVICAL DYSPLASIA

Cervical dysplasias (precancers) are confined to the cervix. They have not yet "learned" to spread to other parts of the body. Early cases are observed. More severe cases are surgically removed. As mentioned in Chapter 1, we recommend the involvement of a gynecologic oncologist for the treatment of cervical cancer. A gynecologic oncologist often manages women with cervical dysplasia. However, because these lesions are precancers and not cancers, patients with cervical dysplasia are usually treated by a primary gynecologist. These physicians receive appropriate training in the treatment of cervical dysplasia and provide excellent care for these lesions.

CERVICAL CANCER

Gynecologic oncologist: There will be many people on your team helping you along this road. The gynecologic oncologist is the "coach" of your team. He or she received training after general obstetrics and gynecology training to become an expert in the medical and surgical management of gynecologic cancers. The gynecologic oncologist will see you first and evaluate your cancer to determine your stage and what treatment options are best for you. This physician will perform surgery if it is needed, and many also will manage chemotherapy if it is needed. Regardless, the gynecologic oncologist will remain involved in your care over the long haul.

Radiation oncologist: This doctor specializes in giving radiation therapy, which is often used to treat cervical cancer. If your gynecologic oncologist determines that you need radiation, you will be referred to a radiation oncologist who will then coordinate your treatment with your gynecologic oncologist.

Medical oncologist: Some gynecologic oncologists do not administer chemotherapy and, if you need it, will work with a medical oncologist who gives the chemotherapy. This doctor will work with your gynecologic and radiation oncologists to coordinate your treatment as a team.

Pathologist: You will likely never meet this doctor, but he or she will examine the tissue from any surgeries or biopsies you have. The pathologist is the person who decides if your biopsy shows cervical dysplasia or cancer. Your pathologist's input will help determine what treatments you will need.

Nurses: You will probably meet several different nurses along this road. There will be nurses in your doctors' offices who will help coordinate your treatment and answer your questions, nurses who will help take care of you in the operating room and after surgery, and nurses who will administer chemotherapy if you need it.

Social worker: Social workers are experts at providing support and helping to find, and use, the resources needed to make it through this process.

YOUR INITIAL APPOINTMENT

Your initial appointment should be with your "coach"— your gynecologic oncologist. This individual will examine you, plan your treatment with you, and be your point person for follow-up.

SCHEDULING

When you call to make your appointment, make sure the person scheduling your initial consultation knows that you are a newly diagnosed cervical cancer patient. You should be seen promptly. Although your condition will certainly seem like a medical emergency, you do not need to be seen the next day. It will often take a week or two to get an appointment. Your cancer has been there for a while, and making sure that everything is arranged correctly is more important than rushing into things. If you begin to feel lost or that things are not moving quickly enough, you can contact the gynecologic oncologist's office or your primary gynecologist office to ask for advice.

Make sure you get exact directions to the office; you will be nervous and won't want to feel frazzled because you are lost and late.

WHAT TO BRING

You should bring any necessary referrals and your insurance information so checking in goes smoothly.

You should also bring copies of previous medical records: pathology reports, colposcopy reports, operative notes, and any radiology reports. Your doctor will also want to see copies of the films from any imaging studies (such as CAT scans) you have had. Your doctor will also want to have the pathologists at his or her hospital review the slides from any biopsies of surgeries you have had. Remember, the more paperwork you have with you, the better. When you call to make the first appointment, you should ask what you can do to provide the doctor with all the information he or she needs.

It is also helpful if you bring a list of any medications you are taking and a list of your medical problems and what surgeries you have had. This information can factor into decisions about your care. Also, when you are nervous, you may forget important details.

WHO TO BRING

You should bring a trusted family member or friend with you. This person can be a source of support for you but also can serve as a scribe. The doctor will provide you with a lot of information, and you will likely feel overwhelmed. When people are stressed, they only retain about 10% of what is said. Your companion can write down the important points and review them with you afterward. This person may also want to bring a tape recorder so you can play back the conversation later; most doctors will be very comfortable with the consultation being voice recorded.

WHAT QUESTIONS TO ASK

You will have lots of questions swimming around in your brain, and having a list can help ensure you get the information you need from your doctor. Here are a few things to ask:

1. What stage do you guesstimate I have based on what you know so far?

2. Do you think I will need surgery or radiation or chemotherapy?

3. What other steps will you take to determine what my treatment will be (such as an exam under anesthesia or CAT scan)?

4. How soon would those evaluations be scheduled?

5. Who will be my contact here if I have questions?

6. Do you have educational materials for me or for my family members, such as my children?

7. Who will coordinate my care? How are subsequent appointments arranged, and when do these happen?

WHAT TESTS NEED TO BE RUN?

Because the treatment of cervical cancer is determined by the stage, staging your cancer will be the first order of business. As discussed in Chapter 1, this requires an outpatient procedure where you receive anesthesia so that your physician can perform a thorough pelvic exam and look into your bladder and rectum. In addition, your doctor will want some basic blood tests to ensure that your kidneys are working normally and to determine if you are anemic. An ECG (electrocardiogram) and a chest X-ray are also usually needed for any procedure requiring anesthesia.

HOW BEST TO CONTACT TEAM MEMBERS

Ask for the best way to contact your doctor should you have any questions or concerns. Usually, there is one contact person in the office you can rely on. Ask how you can get in contact with your doctor in an emergency or after hours.

FINANCIAL IMPLICATIONS OF TREATMENT AND INSURANCE CLEARANCE

Having cancer can cause financial difficulty. It can be especially frustrating and difficult to deal with financial issues when you are so busy concentrating on trying to get well.

If you work outside the home, you will want to figure out how much sick leave you have available and what your options for short- or long-term disability would be.

If you have insurance, you will need to determine what your co-payment requirements are, what referrals you need to be seen by specialists, and what prerequisites there may be before having other procedures. If you need help with these things, ask a social worker to assist you. In some cases, cancer centers and hospitals have financial assistants who can help with these issues as well.

If you don't have health insurance, it is still important to see your gynecologic oncologist; your cancer will only get worse and harder to treat the longer you wait. There are resources available for women who need help and meet certain criteria for financial assistance. Many states have special grants for women with cervical cancer. There are groups that may help provide support with transportation needs and help pay for medications. These programs differ from area to area, so a social worker can help you find out what is available where you live.

Many of these programs are not well advertised, and you will need to find out about them rather than wait and hope they will find out about you. Be assertive in discovering resources to help you through this journey. The organizations listed in Chapter 11 may be able to help.

CHAPTER 3

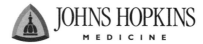

TAKING ACTION—
COMPREHENSIVE TREATMENT
CONSIDERATIONS

OK, your gynecologic oncologist has determined your stage, and it's time to move on to treating your cancer. Cancer can be attacked by three different methods: surgery, chemotherapy, and radiation. Which method, or which combination of methods, is best for you depends on your stage and other aspects of your health (such as whether you still want to have children or are too ill to undergo surgery). Let's talk some more about each of these treatment methods in general.

SURGERY

There are several different surgeries that can be used to treat cervical cancer, depending on the stage.

COLD KNIFE CONE

A cold knife cone involves the removal of part of your cervix. It is a short outpatient procedure that is performed in an operating room so that relaxing medicine can be administered to make you comfortable. The surgery is often performed to remove abnormal cells involving the cervix. With the help of a pathologist, your physician will be able to determine the full extent of the disease. If you only have dysplasia (no evidence of an invasive cancer), a cold knife cone is typically the only procedure you will need. If you have a very early cervical cancer (stage IA1) and want to keep your uterus (because you are hoping to have children), a cold knife cone is also considered to be sufficient surgery. If you have later stage cervical cancer, more treatment will be required. The procedure is usually well tolerated, with low complication rates. You will have some vaginal bleeding for a week or two afterward, and should refrain from having sex for about 4 weeks. There is usually minimal pain, however, and you should feel back to normal in a day or two.

Having a cold knife cone puts you at risk for cervical incompetence (which is when your cervix dilates too soon during pregnancy, potentially causing preterm delivery or miscarriage) or for cervical stenosis (which is when your cervix does not dilate, possibly requiring you to have a cesarean section).

LOOP ELECTROSURGICAL EXCISIONAL PROCEDURE (LEEP)

A loop electrosurgical excisional procedure (LEEP) is often used instead of a cold knife cone for cervical dysplasia. A LEEP is similar to a cold knife cone, except that instead of using a scalpel, the surgeon uses a wire with a current passed through it. A LEEP burns the edges of the tissue, but is thought to heal better than a cold knife cone. Pathologists, the doctors who evaluate the cervix after surgery and make a diagnosis, typically prefer cold knife cone procedures because the cervical margins (edges) are easier to examine. Usually, your physician will recommend a LEEP rather than a cone when there is no evidence of invasion and the lesion involves the outside of the cervix (ectocervix) rather than the inside of the cervix (endocervix).

HYSTERECTOMY

Several different kinds of hysterectomies are available for treating cervical cancer; which one is appropriate depends on your cancer. There is often confusion about what having a "total" or "partial" hysterectomy means, so let's clear that up first: A total hysterectomy means that the cervix and uterus are removed (i.e., the "total" uterus). By contrast, in a supracervical hysterectomy, which is sometimes referred to as a "partial" hysterectomy, only the uterus (and not the cervix) is removed. Clearly a supracervical hysterectomy is not an option for treating cervical cancer! Whether you have your fallopian tubes and ovaries removed is a separate issue. Sometimes people think the terms partial and total refer to whether the ovaries and tubes are removed. This is not the case; you can have a total hysterectomy in which your ovaries are not removed, and you can have a supracervical hysterectomy in which your ovaries are removed.

Total hysterectomies can be done through an incision in your abdominal wall, which is called a total abdominal hysterectomy (TAH). Hysterectomies can also be done vaginally, which is called a total vaginal hysterectomy (TVH). Minimally invasive surgery refers to surgery done with a laparoscope (a camera inserted through your belly button) and may involve robotic assistance in moving the instruments. When a laparoscope is used to help during a vaginal hysterectomy, the procedure is called a laparoscopically assisted vaginal hysterectomy (LAVH). When the hysterectomy is done entirely with the laparoscope, the procedure is called a total laparoscopic hysterectomy (TLH). Which procedure is right for you depends on many factors, including how big your uterus is, how much you weigh, how many other surgeries you have had, and if you have had children vaginally. Total hysterectomies are used for cervical cancer when the cancer is at a very early stage (stage IA1) and you are not planning on having any more children. Occasionally, it is done for later stage cancers after you have had radiation.

If you have a hysterectomy, your doctor will also talk with you about whether to remove your fallopian tubes and ovaries (called a bilateral salpingo-oopherectomy). If you have already gone through menopause, you should have your tubes and ovaries removed at the time of your surgery. If you have not gone through menopause, you should discuss this more with your doctor because removing your tubes and ovaries will cause you to begin menopause. Although cervical cancer could have spread to your ovaries, the risk of this is small. The main reason for removing your ovaries is to protect you from developing ovarian cancer and to prevent you from needing surgery for any cysts that develop in your ovaries in the future. Also, if you need radiation after surgery for your cervical cancer, it will likely cause your ovaries to stop working and you would begin menopause anyway.

Radical hysterectomies are extra large (outsized) total hysterectomies. A total hysterectomy removes just the cervix and uterus and leaves all the supporting tissue behind. A radical hysterectomy removes the cervix and uterus but also removes part or all of the ligaments that hold the cervix in place. This surgery can be done with or without a bilateral salpingo-oopherectomy. Radical hysterectomies are traditionally performed by an incision through the abdomen. However, more and more doctors are now performing these procedures with minimally invasive surgery using a laparoscope, usually with the assistance of a robot.

In a radical hysterectomy, the doctor removes more tissue around the cervix in order to get better margins around the cancer and to improve the chance that the cancer will *not* come back. Radical hysterectomies are typically performed for stage I cervical cancers. Because your doctor has to remove more tissue and your bladder is right next to your cervix, this surgery can irritate your bladder, and you will need to have a catheter (often called a Foley catheter) for at least 3 days and often for up to 2 weeks after the surgery. You can go home with the catheter, and the nurses will show you how to take care of it. Radical hysterectomy is fairly well tolerated, but it is major surgery and you will feel sore and tired for several weeks afterward.

After any hysterectomy, you should not have sex for at least 4 weeks. There is a small risk (about 1%) of developing a fistula (an abnormal opening) between your bladder and vagina or between one of your ureters (the tubes from your kidney to your bladder) and vagina. These fistulas result in urine leaking out the vagina. In the rare case this happens, surgery is often required to fix the problem.

TRACHELECTOMY

In a trachelectomy, the entire cervix is removed but the uterus is left in place. A radical trachelectomy is only done if your cervical cancer is stage IA2 or IB1 (in other words, small and still just in your cervix) and you want to have children. A radical trachelectomy is similar to a radical hysterectomy in that the cervix and part or all of the ligaments that hold it in place are removed. However, in a radical trachelectomy, the body of the uterus is kept in place and reconnected to the vagina. This procedure is relatively new, and it is unclear if there is more risk of recurrence if a woman has a radical trachelectomy versus a radical hysterectomy. As mentioned above, the advantage of a radical trachelectomy is that the patient can still get pregnant and carry the baby to term. However since the cervix's job is to keep your baby in the uterus until it opens (dilates) at delivery, having a radical trachelectomy puts you at risk for preterm delivery. A stitch, called a cerclage, is placed in the bottom of the uterus to help keep it closed, and a cesarean section is needed to deliver the baby.

LYMPH NODE DISSECTION

Infection-fighting cells use a sort of "highway" called the lymph system to move throughout your body. The highway connects small bumps throughout your body called lymph nodes. These lymph nodes serve as rest stations where the infection-fighting cells can hang out. Unfortunately, cancer cells can sometimes get onto that highway system and use it to travel through the body. If this happens, they often stay in the lymph nodes. Lymph node dissections can be done through an incision in your abdomen or with a minimally invasive approach using the laparoscope with or without robot assistance, depending on what other procedures you are having done at the same time. If you are having a radical hysterectomy or radical trachelectomy, your doctor will also remove the lymph nodes in your pelvis and sometimes along the aorta to determine if cancer cells have gotten into the lymph nodes. Sometimes if you are having radiation without a hysterectomy, your doctor will also do a lymph node dissection to help determine how extensively the cancer has spread. A lymph node dissection usually is well tolerated. The risks of a lymph node dissection include injury to the blood vessels or nerves that are near the lymph nodes. Also, some women develop lymphedema, a condition in which the lymph fluid builds up in the legs causing swelling.

EXENTERATION

Exenteration is very extensive surgery that is sometimes done for recurrent cervical cancer. It is rarely done for a newly diagnosed cervical cancer. This surgery is so extensive that it is typically only done if there is a possibility that it could lead to a cure. Because the risks and side effects of this surgery are greater than with most surgeries, you and your doctor need to have a detailed discussion about the goals and outcomes before moving forward. There are several types of exenterations. In all of the procedures, the vagina, uterus, and cervix, if present, are removed. Often a new vagina can be created from your skin or muscles (called "flaps"). A total exenteration also involves removing the bladder and rectum. With an anterior exenteration, the vagina and bladder are removed, but the rectum is left in place. With a posterior exenteration, the vagina and rectum are removed, but the bladder is left in place.

A pouch is then created to make a new bladder, which either requires you to catheterize yourself or to wear an ostomy bag to collect your urine. Another pouch (called a colostomy), which requires an ostomy bag, is often created to collect your stool. However, sometimes the colon is put back together and a colostomy is not required.

RADIATION

Radiation is often used to treat cervical cancer. It can be used as the main treatment or in addition to surgery (either before or after). Radiation comes in two forms: external beam and brachytherapy. Radiation can be given with a small dose of weekly chemotherapy, which is called chemosensitization.

EXTERNAL BEAM

In external beam radiation, the radiation oncologist directs radiation at your cancer from outside your body. The radiation oncologist will first take a CAT scan to carefully measure exactly where to aim the radiation. He or she will then tattoo small blue dots to your skin to mark where to give you the radiation for each treatment. You will receive a treatment daily over several weeks (usually about 5 to 6 weeks), but each treatment itself is very short (usually less than 10 minutes). Most women feel fatigued while receiving radiation. It can cause irritation to the skin as well as the bladder or bowels, sometimes leading to blood in the urine or diarrhea. Radiation can make your vagina stenotic (tightened), and you may need to use dilators to keep your vagina open. Often, radiation is given with a type of chemotherapy called Platinol AQ (cisplatin), which helps the radiation work better (chemosensitization).

BRACHYTHERAPY

In brachytherapy, the radiation oncologist puts radiation inside your body for a short period of time. It is often given after external beam radiation. If the radiation is being given as primary treatment without surgery and the uterus is still in place, the radiation is placed directly in the uterus and the vagina using small radioactive rods, thus allowing the radiation oncologist to put a lot of radiation where the cancer is located (the cervix). This procedure typically requires at least one trip to the operating room. The radiation is given over about two to three treatment sessions. If your uterus has already been removed and your physician has recommended radiation, the radiation is given to the top of the vagina after the external beam radiation. Once again, about two to three treatment sessions are required.

There are two ways to give the brachytherapy, called low-dose rate and high-dose rate. Because high-dose rate brachytherapy is faster, the radiation can be given over a shorter period of time. It does not usually require admission to the hospital. However, there is not as much experience with high-dose rate treatment and it is not available at every cancer center. Both types require one or more tubes to be placed next to the tissue that needs the radiation. The radiation is then placed into the tube and the tissue receives the appropriate dose of radiation. Usually two or more treatments or sessions are required. Most times the placement of the tube requires a trip to the operating room, but sometimes with high-dose rate radiation the tube can be placed in the radiation oncology treatment area rather than the operating room. This is one of the factors that can make high-dose rate radiation more convenient. As mentioned high-dose rate is faster than low-dose rate radiation. With low-dose rate radiation, you will stay in the hospital on bed rest for a day or two, until the doctors remove the beads and the form. While you are on bed rest, you will need to stay very still and will only be able to have visitors for a very short period of time. With high-dose rate radiation, the treatment is given for only a short time (typically less than 30 minutes) and can therefore be given as an outpatient procedure without admission to the hospital.

CHEMOTHERAPY

Chemotherapy involves the use of drugs to treat cancer. The medication is often given in the vein (intravenously), but is sometimes given by mouth. Chemotherapy is used in two different ways for cervical cancer. The chemotherapy can either be given with another treatment or by itself.

Chemotherapy can be given with radiation therapy in order to make your cells more susceptible to the radiation so that the radiation works better. This approach is called chemosensitization. Platinol AQ is the most common chemotherapy drug used for this.

Surgery and/or radiation are used as the primary treatment(s) for cervical cancer that remains limited to the pelvis. Once the disease has spread beyond the pelvis, there is too much disease to treat appropriately with surgery or radiation. Therefore, chemotherapy is given by itself if your cancer has metastasized (spread) outside of your pelvis (for example, to your lungs). Chemotherapy works throughout the body. Although dramatic responses are sometimes seen, it is very unusual for chemotherapy to make metastatic cancer go away forever.

For metastatic cervical cancer, the combination of two chemotherapy drugs appears more effective than one drug by itself. Currently, a platinum drug such as Platinol AQ or Paraplatin (carboplatin) is given with a second drug. Paraplatin and Taxol (paclitaxel) are a common combination used as the first chemotherapy regimen against cervical cancer. For this chemotherapy, you receive intravenous infusions as an outpatient every 3 weeks for 6 cycles. Chemotherapy can produce many side effects, which are discussed in detail in Chapter 4. Briefly, chemotherapy makes most women feel tired. Many women experience nausea with chemotherapy, but there are many new medications that can help relieve this side effect. Often, your appetite will decrease for the week after you receive your infusion. This type of chemotherapy makes you lose your hair, but it will grow back after you are finished with the treatments. This combination of chemotherapy can also cause tingling and numbness in your toes and fingers (peripheral neuropathy).

There are other chemotherapy regimens that your doctor may recommend if your cancer recurs or worsens. Each type of chemotherapy has its own side effects, and you should talk with your doctor about what to expect with the particular type of chemotherapy you will be receiving.

CLINICAL TRIALS

Clinical trails are how we make medical care better. Without them, medical care would never improve. Clinical trials try to answer all sorts of questions: Is there a better way to screen for a disease? Is there a way to prevent the disease? Is there a safe way to treat early disease that involves less treatment? Are there better surgeries we can perform? Better ways to give radiation? Better chemotherapy? Are there new drugs that would be effective against recurrent disease? Are there new medicines we can give to help with side effects? Are there other things we can do (support groups, acupuncture, etc.) to help with side effects? All these questions and many more have been asked in clinical trials and will continue to be asked as we try to improve cancer care.

Clinical trials of new drugs or treatments are designed in different phases, depending on what type of question they are trying to answer. Phase I trials are for new drugs or treatments and aim to find out if a drug might work and how much of it can be given safely. Usually only a small number of patients are in these studies. Phase I studies are typically for women whose cancer has not responded to other treatments.

Phase II studies seek to determine if a treatment works against the cancer. They examine whether patients' cancer stops growing or even decreases with the drug and whether side effects occur. These trials are larger than Phase I trials, but usually involve less than 50 patients. These trials are typically for women whose cancer is no longer responding to the treatments or drugs currently available.

Phase III trials try to determine if a new drug, a different combination of drugs, or a new treatment works better than current treatments (also called the "standard of care"). In order to determine whether there is a difference, more women need to be treated with both options, so these studies are larger. Patients are usually randomized (like flipping a coin) to one treatment or another. The randomization may be "blind" so that neither the patient nor their doctors know which treatment they are receiving. This "blind" approach helps make sure no favoritism (bias) sneaks in that would falsely make one of the treatments look better or worse than it really is. These studies examine whether a treatment leads to fewer recurrences, longer survival, better quality of life, and fewer side effects.

Other clinical studies try to answer different questions about how to improve cancer care. For example, a study may focus on whether a type of imaging is effective at locating cancer in your body, or a study may consider whether certain types of counseling help improve quality of life during treatment.

Often clinical trials, especially for new drugs and treatments, are run nationally and directed by the National Cancer Institute (NCI) or the Gynecologic Oncology Group (GOG).

If you are interested in participating in a clinical trial, you should ask your doctor if any are appropriate for you. Likewise, your doctor may ask if you would like to participate in a clinical trail. Before beginning any trial, make sure you understand what is involved. Below are several questions to ask yourself in deciding if you want to participate in a study:

What is the purpose of the study?

What does the study involve? What kind of tests and treatment will I have?

How are treatments given, and what side effects might I expect?

What are the risks and benefits?

How long will the study last?

Will I incur any costs? Will my insurance company pay for part of this?

When will the results be known?

A particular clinical trial may not help you. If we knew for sure that the treatment being tested worked better than the other options, then we wouldn't need to do a trial! Nonetheless, clinical trials help medical care grow, and many women feel better knowing they contributed to improving cancer care for other women down the line.

WHAT TREATMENT CAN I EXPECT?

OK, so now you have a general sense of what the options are for treating cervical cancer. But you are probably most concerned about what treatment YOU will receive! The appropriate treatment for cervical cancer depends a lot on your stage and also on other individual factors, such as your general health. In general, earlier cancer is treated with surgery, and later cancer is treated with radiation.

STAGE O (CARCINOMA IN SITU)

Stage o disease or carcinoma in situ is a noninvasive disease. A cold knife cone or a LEEP is usually all that is necessary. These surgeries not only confirm the diagnosis but are also considered sufficient treatment. Occasionally, especially in a woman who has had multiple cold knife cones and/or LEEPs, a hysterectomy is recommended because a cold knife cone can not be performed safely. As with cervical cancer, there is always a chance that even if all the disease is removed it can come back, and you will need to continue to get PAP smears after your surgery.

STAGE IA1

This is the earliest stage of cancer, in which there is only a microscopic amount of disease on your cervix. If you are planning on having children in the future, a cold knife cone should be sufficient treatment. If you do not plan to have any more children, a total hysterectomy is recommended.

STAGE IA2

In this stage, the cancer is still microscopic and only on your cervix, but it is a tiny bit bigger than in stage IA1. There is some risk, although still small, that the cancer could have spread outside of your cervix. Therefore, more surgery is needed. Usually a radical hysterectomy and lymph node dissection are performed. If you are planning to have children in the future, a trachelectomy with lymph node dissection may be done instead.

STAGE IB1

In this stage, the cancer is smaller than 4 cm and is still only on your cervix as far as the doctor can tell in the exam under anesthesia. Usually a radical hysterectomy and lymph node dissection are performed. If having children in the future is very important to you, it may be possible to have a trachelectomy and lymph node dissection, but it will depend on the size of the cancer. Radiation can also be used to treat this stage of cancer and has equal cure rates.

STAGE IB2

In this stage, the cancer is more than 4 cm but is still only on the cervix. Here treatment recommendations depend more on each individual case. Sometimes a radical hysterectomy and lymph node dissection can be done. Other times, radiation with Platinol AQ chemosensitization can be given. There are risks and benefits to either approach, but they both appear to work equally well. Surgery is associated with immediate problems such as blood loss, but long-term problems are not as frequent. Surgery is completed in just a few hours. Radiation, on the other hand, does not have as many immediate side effects but causes long-term issues such as scarring and shortening of the vagina, which can make sex difficult or painful, and can cause pain while urinating and difficulty with bowel movements.

The problem with performing a radical hysterectomy for this stage of cancer is that radiation may be necessary afterward. Radiation is given after surgery to "clean up" if there are positive margins (cancer cells found in the edge of the cut tissue), positive parametrial tissue (cancer cells in the tissue that was removed but was next to the cervix), or positive lymph nodes (cancer cells in the lymph nodes). This radiation is given to eliminate any cancer cells that surgery did not remove and helps reduce the risk of recurrence. In general, doctors avoid doing radical surgery followed by radiation because it tends to lead to high rates of side effects. You should talk with your doctor about the pros and cons of each approach in your particular case.

STAGE IIA—IIIB

These more advanced stages are usually treated first with radiation and Platinol AQ chemosensitization because the chance that you will need radiation after surgery is very high and having radiation alone works just as well with fewer complications.

STAGE IV

In stage IV, the cancer has spread outside of your pelvis, and local treatments, like surgery or radiation, will not be enough. Therefore, chemotherapy is the best treatment. Usually two drugs such as Paraplatin and Taxol are used together. Sometimes surgery or radiation may also be recommended to treat your symptoms, such as severe vaginal bleeding or pain.

CHAPTER 4

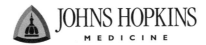

BEING PREPARED— THE SIDE EFFECTS OF TREATMENT

B y now you and your doctor have probably sat down and come up with a treatment plan. It may be reassuring to have a course of attack against your cancer, but you are probably starting to wonder how the treatment will affect you. Each type of treatment we use to combat cervical cancer (surgery, radiation, and chemotherapy) carries its own side effects and complications, and we'll talk about what you can expect with each of these, along with some strategies to prevent or minimize side effects. It is also important to remember that each woman's cancer is different, as is her reaction to treatment.

Before talking about specifics of each therapy, let's address some concerns that are common to all forms of cervical cancer treatment, namely their impact on you as a woman in terms of sexuality, childbearing, and menopause.

First off, your cervix is probably not something you talked about on a daily basis before. Many women are uncomfortable talking about their female organs and now, all of a sudden, you will be thinking and talking about them a lot. Some women feel dirty or embarrassed about having cervical cancer. It is important to move beyond this. You don't have to discuss every detail with everyone, but feelings of shame are not going to help you deal with your cancer and may keep you from getting the support from others you deserve and need.

It is also important to talk with your partner about how your diagnosis will affect your sex life. Cervical cancer itself may make sex difficult, since vaginal intercourse can cause bleeding or pain. After surgery you should not have sex for at least 4–6 weeks (until the doctor examines you and says you are healed). Surgery may shorten the length of your vagina. Radiation can cause scarring and thinning of the vaginal walls, making intercourse more difficult. Using dilators and vaginal creams can help keep the vagina open after radiation. Exploring different positions may help, given the changes in your anatomy. It is also important to remember that there are many other ways to express love and experience sexual pleasure such as dancing, cuddling, petting, and oral stimulation. While it may be difficult to talk about these issues with your partner, it is better to have a frank discussion rather than remain silent.

Another issue that a woman newly diagnosed with cervical cancer may face regardless of the treatment she receives is loss of fertility. If you have not completed your childbearing, especially if you do not have any children yet, the diagnosis of cervical cancer can be especially hard. You may have to cope with the possibility of not being able to have children on top of dealing with the treatment of your cancer. If your cervical cancer is early, your doctor may be able to do a more limited surgery (a cone or a trachelectomy) that preserves your ability to have children. If your cancer is more advanced, however, these procedures are not enough to appropriately fight your cancer. While your doctor understands the important desire to preserve your fertility, this goal must be balanced, if possible, against the objective of adequately treating and curing the cancer. Support groups can be a good resource to help you through this loss, and friends and family members also can be sources of support. After you have fought your cancer, adoption may be an option.

Treatment may also bring about menopause if you have not already begun it. Surgery may include removing your ovaries if you are close to menopause or there is concern that the cancer may have spread to them. Radiation can also lead to menopause because your ovaries will be irradiated (although if you require radiation, your physician can, in certain situations, perform an oophoropexy in which the ovaries are moved out of the pelvis and into the abdomen. This places them outside of the area to be irradiated and allows the patient to maintain ovarian function and can allow for collection of eggs at a later date for in vitro fertilization).

Menopause is different for each woman. Symptoms can include hot flashes, vaginal dryness, decreased libido (interest in sex), urinary incontinence (leaking some urine when you cough or sneeze), or memory problems. Other health effects include an increased risk of heart disease and strokes and loss of bone strength.

There is a lot of literature about hormone replacement, and while doctors previously thought it was a great idea for protection of your heart and bones, some of that enthusiasm has been tempered by recent studies suggesting that hormone replacement therapy carries increased risks of heart disease, stroke, blood clots, and breast cancer. However, hormone replacement after entering surgery- or radiation-induced menopause is a little different. Basically, it gives you back the hormones you would have had normally, before you received a treatment. Therefore, we believe hormone replacement should be as safe as if you continued to have your ovaries functioning as normal. It is important to talk with your doctor about whether your ovaries will be affected by your treatment, and if so, whether hormone replacement therapy is a good idea for you.

With those issues under your belt, let's turn to what you can expect based on the treatment you receive.

SURGERY

POSTOPERATIVE ISSUES

A radical hysterectomy is major surgery. You will usually spend 2–5 days in the hospital postoperatively and will feel very tired and sore afterward. Once you can eat and walk around and are on oral pain medications, you will be able to go home. You should expect to feel sore and not quite up to normal functioning for a few weeks. You should not drive while you are on narcotics, and even afterward, you should not drive until you feel you can do so safely. Narcotics can cause constipation, so you should take stool softeners while you are on them. Narcotics can also make you itchy, and taking Benadryl or switching to a different narcotic can help. It is important to keep up with your pain. Take your pain medications on a schedule before your pain becomes too much. It is much harder to rein pain back in than to keep it well controlled in the first place. The same is true for nausea. Anesthesia and narcotics make some women nauseous, but there are many medications that can help. Ask your doctor for them if you are experiencing nausea.

Each woman recovers from surgery differently. It is a good idea to recruit friends and family to help out when you get home from the hospital. You will be able to walk up and down steps and shower, but you will likely feel exhausted and sore for some time. When to return to work is also an individual decision, depending on how you are recovering and what type of work you do. Most women take 4–6 weeks off after a radical hysterectomy.

If you have a laparoscopic or robotic surgery, the recovery time is much shorter, and you will usually be able to go home the day after surgery and return to work much more rapidly.

Regardless of whether your surgery is open or laparoscopic, the top of your vagina needs time to heal. Thus it is important to not have sex until your doctor has examined you and said it is OK.

After surgery, you will have a catheter in your bladder. You will probably have to keep it in for at least 3 days postoperatively and sometimes up to 14 days. Radical hysterectomies disrupt some of the nerve connections to your bladder, which can lead to your bladder not emptying correctly. The catheter allows your bladder to rest and recover its normal function. Instead of a Foley catheter (constant catheterization), some centers have the patient catheterize herself several times a day (intermittent catheterization). This method allows the patient to get around without a bag but requires more work on the patient's part.

Sometimes after the catheter is removed, patients have difficulty urinating. If so, you may need the catheter reinserted and left in for a few more days. Don't worry, it is incredibly rare for your bladder not to recover its normal function; sometimes it just takes time.

RARE COMPLICATIONS

Your doctor will talk with you about some possible long-term complications that can develop after surgery. This is not done to scare you; rather, it is part of the process called "informed consent" so that you know what is about to happen to you and the possible implications of proceeding with or declining treatment.

If your lymph nodes are removed during your surgery, there is a risk of developing lymphedema in one or both legs. Lymphedema is a condition in which the lymph fluid that normally drains out of your legs accumulates in your legs because the channels back into your body are blocked. It is treated by wrapping your legs, thus reducing swelling by forcing the fluid out of your lower extremities.

Anytime you have surgery, there is a risk of forming adhesions. Normally, organs in the abdomen and pelvis are separate. However, surgery can cause inflammation that can result in bands of scar tissue being created between the pelvic and abdominal organs. This scar tissue is referred to as adhesions. Adhesions can cause the intestines to become stuck to the uterus and/or the ovaries. The effects of adhesions can be worse if you require radiation after surgery. Adhesions can pinch off your bowels, leading to a bowel obstruction. When bowel obstructions occur, you become very nauseated, vomit frequently, and are unable to have bowel movements. Another surgery is sometimes needed to correct this blockage.

Because radical hysterectomies require removal of tissue right next to the bladder, there is a risk of developing a fistula (an abnormal passageway between two organs in the body or between an organ and the exterior of the body) from your vagina into the bladder (called a vesicovaginal fistula). Fistulas happen more frequently if you need radiation after surgery, and they usually require another surgery to repair.

As explained previously, exenterations are very extensive. They are usually done when recurrent cervical cancer is confined to the top of the vagina and the surgery provides a hope for a cure. The surgery requires the vagina be removed, and a new vagina is often created out of skin or muscles from another part of your body.

Additionally, exenterations usually involve removing your bladder and/or rectum. If your bladder is removed, your doctor will create a new bladder from your intestines. Sometimes a new bladder that has an opening onto your skin can be created, which you will need to catheterize several times a day. Other times, the new bladder will empty directly into a bag attached to your stomach. If the rectum is removed, your doctor will create a colostomy, where your intestines empty into a bag on your stomach. Nurses will help you learn how to care for these ostomies, and support groups are available to help you adjust to your changed body.

RADIATION

EARLY EFFECTS

Radiation causes some changes in your body (acute side effects) while you are undergoing treatments. Although these can be very troubling, they usually resolve soon after the treatments are completed.

Your skin can become irritated, similar to a sunburn. Your radiation oncologist can suggest or prescribe creams to ease this symptom.

Radiation aimed at your pelvis can affect your bladder, causing radiation cystitis (inflammation in your bladder), which can make you feel like you have to urinate frequently. It can also affect your bowels, leading to more frequent stools and sometimes diarrhea.

Additionally, you will likely feel very tired during treatments. Having friends and family members help you with tasks around the house is a good idea. Because the treatments are every day for several weeks, scheduling will be an important consideration. Treatments are usually reasonably quick, and the radiation oncology staff will try their best to minimize the disruptions to your daily activities caused by radiation therapy.

LATER EFFECTS

Radiation can cause long-term changes (chronic side effects) in your body. Your skin may remain sensitive for quite a while, and the lining of your vagina will likely become thinner as well. Radiation can lead to vaginal stenosis (where the vagina becomes smaller and shorter). Using estrogen cream and dilators can help prevent this, and using a personal lubricant can help combat vaginal dryness and make sex more enjoyable.

Radiation can affect your bowels and bladder long term. Rarely, radiation cystitis can continue or develop after treatments are complete, which can lead to frequent urination or blood in your urine. Medications can help control the bladder irritation. Radiation proctitis refers to inflammation in your colon and rectum caused by the radiation. It can lead to diarrhea or blood in your stools. It is important to let your doctors know if you develop blood in your stools or urine so they can make sure it is due to radiation and not something else.

As mentioned in the surgical complications section, radiation coupled with surgery increases your risk of developing adhesions, which can cause bowel blockages. Sometimes another surgery is necessary to release these adhesions. Also, radiation after surgery increases your risk of developing fistulas (abnormal connections) between your bladder and vagina. Another surgery is usually needed to close off these connections.

CHEMOTHERAPY

As discussed in Chapter 3, chemotherapy is given in two ways for cervical cancer: to help radiation work better (chemosensitization), and as a treatment by itself. In general, chemosensitization with low amounts of Platinol AQ is very well tolerated. Chemotherapy with Paraplatin and Taxol is more intensive, but with support most women are able to get through all 6 cycles without too much difficulty.

Chemotherapy with Platinol AQ or Paraplatin and Taxol can make you feel tired. Chemotherapy can cause nausea and vomiting, but there are medicines to help prevent these symptoms. If nausea is a problem for you during chemotherapy, let your doctor know so he or she can give you stronger antinausea medications. Also, eating small but more frequent meals can be helpful. Avoiding spicy or strong-smelling foods can decrease nausea. Something bland, like crackers or liquids can often help settle your stomach. Some women find peppermints or ginger candies helpful as well.

Most women will have decreased energy levels and lower appetite while they are receiving their chemotherapy. Some women experience constipation as well.

Most women do not lose their hair while they are receiving Platinol AQ. However, Taxol usually causes hair loss. Hair loss can be very difficult for some women. Your hair may be an important part of how you see yourself as a woman. There are several different ways to cope with hair loss. Some women get a wig. If you plan on getting a wig, you may want to do so before you lose your hair so it can be matched to your natural hair color. Some insurance companies cover wigs for chemotherapy patients. Check to see if your plan covers a "skull prosthesis for side effects of cancer treatment." Hair loss usually starts between 10 and 14 days after your first chemotherapy infusion. Some women shave their heads before their hair falls out so they will feel more in charge. Assembling a collection of scarves and hats is a good idea. Asking friends and family members to find you unique head coverings can be a way for you to involve them.

Platinol AQ and Paraplatin can affect the nerves that go to your hands and feet, and you may develop tingling in your fingers and toes. This symptom usually improves slowly after the chemotherapy is completed but can lead to long-term decreased feeling and coordination. Platinol AQ can also cause kidney toxicity. This may cause your kidneys to have difficulty with their usual functions of making urine and getting rid of waste. Intravenous fluid (hydration) is usually given to reduce the odds of this happening.

Chemotherapy can also make you feel more befuddled than usual; sometimes this effect is referred to as "chemo brain." Try to be tolerant of yourself, knowing that you might be more forgetful than usual. Often making lists can help keep you organized and on track.

Many women continue to work while they are receiving chemotherapy; however, everyone's experience is different, and your ability to work will depend on how you tolerate chemotherapy and what kind of work you do.

Chemotherapy can also lower your blood cells. There are three types of blood cells: white blood cells, red blood cells, and platelets. If your red blood cells are low, you are anemic. Usually anemia is not a problem, although it may make you feel more tired than usual. If your red blood cell levels get very low during chemotherapy, you may need an injection such as Procrit (epoetin alfa) or Aranesp (darbepoetin alfa) to help keep your red blood cells up. If your levels get very low, you may require a blood transfusion, which can usually be done as an outpatient procedure in the infusion center where you receive your chemotherapy. Blood transfusions are generally safe, and the risk of getting an infection such as hepatitis or HIV is very low.

Chemotherapy can also decrease your white blood cells. These cells fight off infections. If your white blood cells are too low, you are at risk of developing infections. You may have to take antibiotics to protect against infections. It is also very important to notify your doctor if you develop a fever while you are on chemotherapy, as this can be a sign of a serious infection. If your white blood cells are low after chemotherapy, you may need a shot of Neulasta (pegfilgrastim) to help keep them elevated with your next cycle of chemotherapy.

Platelets are like the Band-Aids of your blood—they form clots to stop bleeding if you cut or scrape yourself. Usually, having low platelets does not cause serious problems, but if they are too low, your next cycle of chemotherapy might need to be delayed.

While this chapter contains lots of information that may sound discouraging, it is important to remember it is intended as a list of side effects that COULD happen and is designed to help you anticipate and cope with any problems that come up. Most women recover well from surgery, get through radiation, and complete their chemotherapy with minimal side effects.

CHAPTER 5

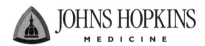

STRAIGHT TALK— COMMUNICATION WITH FAMILY, FRIENDS, AND COWORKERS

B y now you know your diagnosis and stage and have a treatment strategy mapped out. As you absorb this information, you will need to begin telling those around you about your diagnosis.

Talking about your diagnosis and treatment can be difficult—you are likely not used to talking to people about your cervix! Everyone has different levels of comfort with their body, and what level of detail you want to provide will depend on both your own level of comfort and who you are talking to. There are two separate groups of people: those you want to tell (your friends and family, who will be your main sources of support) and those you have to tell (your boss and other people whose jobs will be affected by your treatment).

One of the most important family members to speak with is your partner. Health problems, especially serious ones such as cancer, can shake up even rock-solid relationships. The way people see each other can change when roles and self-image are upended by a cancer diagnosis. Suddenly you may need much more support, both emotionally and physically. Daily routines will be disrupted. Facing a serious health crisis may make you reflect and question past decisions. And, as discussed earlier, the diagnosis and treatment can significantly alter your sexual relationship. All these feelings and changes are natural, but honest, open communication will be important.

You will also need to speak with your children. The conversation you have with your kids will clearly depend on how old they are. Even very young children will sense that something is wrong with their mother, and lying to them will only create distrust and make them more frightened. While young children may not understand what cancer is, they can understand that you are sick and that you need to see doctors to help you feel better. Playacting can help children deal with your treatment. Sometimes children are concerned that they can "catch" cancer, so reassure them that they and other members of your family will not get sick because you are.

Teenagers' reactions can vary. They may be very supportive and helpful one day, and the next day, they may seem selfish and act like your illness was designed specifically to torture them. It is important to remember that they still need to be able to be teenagers and that "acting out" usually reflects their concern for you. Talk with them and let them know that although you will need them to help out more than usual, you want to make sure they have some time for themselves, too.

Adult children may have difficulty dealing with your illness, as it may make them realize that they, and you, are getting older. Roles may change if you now need to rely on them to help take care of you. This can be rather disconcerting for both parties, but being aware of this dynamic can help ease some of the tension that may arise.

Talking with your parents can be difficult. Often they will feel like they should have been the one diagnosed with cancer instead of you. They will want to help you, so try to have some things prepared that they can help you with. Your parents may become significantly more active in your life again because you need help. Old roles and habits can be comforting in times of strain. However, reverting to childhood roles can reactivate some conflicts. It is important to talk with your parents about how they can help support you as an adult, not you as a child.

Your parents may also have personal experience dealing with illness or even cancer. Talking with them about how they have managed health problems can be an enlightening and helpful process for you both.

Your siblings and other family members will also be worried about you. Family dynamics can be strained by an illness. Consider appointing one person to be the information source and distribute information to everyone else. Doing so can help you avoid having to repeat information to multiple family members while also averting family disputes that may arise if some individuals feel you are telling others more than you are telling them.

Talking with friends is important as well. They can be a huge source of support for you. Many will want to help you in a concrete way, and it can be useful to have a list of tasks you need help with (such as transportation to radiation treatments or watching the kids for a bit so you can nap as you recover from surgery). On the other hand, some friends may not call after they hear the news; they are worried about you but may not know what to say. Don't be shy—let them know you need their care and support. They will likely be relieved that there is something concrete they can do for you. Consider getting a list of email addresses and sending out periodic updates, thus reducing the burden of informing many different people while also allowing your friends to help each other support you.

What to tell your boss and coworkers can be difficult as well. By law, you are not required to tell them any specifics about your diagnosis or prognosis. However, you will need to inform your boss that you are ill and will need time off or accommodations to allow for your treatments. Each person and workplace is different, so how much you tell your coworkers and boss will depend on your particular situation. Keep in mind that coworkers can be a good source of support and may be able to pitch in and help at work as you go through treatment. The Americans with Disabilities Act provides some job protections so that you or your family members can take time off from work if necessary (http://www.ada.gov).

CHAPTER 6

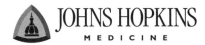

Maintaining Balance—
Work and Life During
Treatment

M ost likely, when you heard you had cancer, your world seemed to tilt off kilter, and everything seemed different. It can be very strange to realize that other aspects of your life progress as if nothing has changed. You should certainly take time coming to grips with your diagnosis and allow yourself leeway to feel sad or even to cry seemingly out of the blue on some days. However, re-engaging in normal life activities is not only necessary, it can make you feel better and more like yourself again.

How much your treatment will impact your day-to-day activities depends largely on what treatments you receive.

If you are having surgery, the disruption in your routine will happen right away. For a hysterectomy, you will probably need to take time off work. After most hysterectomies, you should expect to spend from 2 to 4 days in the hospital. Once you go home, you will still not feel quite yourself and should not be driving or doing heavy lifting. The surgery section in Chapter 4 discusses these postsurgical considerations, as well as catheterization, which may also delay your return to work. Depending on the demands of your job, you can expect to need between 2 and 6 weeks off. If your surgery will be done robotically, you can expect a much faster recovery; usually you can go home the next morning and will feel back to normal much sooner.

Some women want to return to work as soon as possible so they can feel more like themselves again and think about something besides their cancer. Other women want as much time as possible to get themselves in order prior to returning to work. The Family and Medical Leave Act of 1993 provides some protection for you to take time off work while you are recovering.

Other responsibilities you might have (such as raising children) do not provide medical leave. It is important to arrange for help with these tasks, especially during the first few days after you come home from the hospital.

If you are having radiation, the disruption to your schedule will be less per day but will be spread over a longer period of time. Radiation is given in short treatments every day over several weeks. Most radiation oncology centers are set up to get patients in and out quickly in an attempt to minimize the impact on their schedule. You will likely need to work with your boss to align your work schedule so you can attend your radiation appointments. While some women have to take time off from work during their radiation treatments, most find it possible to work during radiation.

Radiation usually is well tolerated but tends to make you tired. Expect to have less energy than usual. Asking friends and family to help you around the house or with childcare during this time is a good idea.

The impact of chemotherapy on your daily routine depends on which chemotherapy regimen you receive. Platinol AQ chemosensitization is usually fairly well tolerated, but it will require a weekly infusion in addition to your radiation appointments.

Other chemotherapies are given on different schedules. These schedules are called "cycles." In general, you will receive an infusion of chemotherapy on the first day of a cycle and have other appointments or tasks on other days. For instance, you may receive chemotherapy on day 1, come back for some lab work to make sure your blood levels are OK on day 5, have another infusion of chemotherapy on day 8, and have your blood work checked a few other days. This cycle would then repeat itself after 21 or 28 days.

Often you can have your blood work done at a lab near your house if you live farther away from the hospital. On the days you have chemotherapy, you will usually come to the infusion center. Some infusion centers are set up as open areas so patients can share their experiences and gain strength from each other, while others are set up to focus more on providing a quiet, private space. Usually the infusion process takes a few hours, so you should come prepared. Consider bringing a friend with you, especially for the first few sessions until you know what to expect.

The side effects of each type of chemotherapy are different, so it is important to speak with your doctor or chemotherapy nurse about what to expect. In general, if you are going to experience gastrointestinal problems, symptoms usually start between 16 and 48 hours after you receive the chemotherapy. Chemotherapy can make you feel tired and decrease your appetite; allow yourself some downtime to take naps and indulge in the foods you do crave.

While receiving chemotherapy, your white blood cells (the cells that are in charge of fighting off infection) can decrease significantly. This usually happens about 1 week after your infusion. When your counts are low, it is especially important to avoid infection. Wash your hands often, stay away from sick people, and consider wearing a mask if you have to travel by plane during those times. Receiving a flu shot before you start chemotherapy is also a good idea.

Regardless of what treatments you receive, it is important to let your friends and family help you. Make a list of tasks you could use some assistance with so when people ask if there is anything they can do, you can say, "Why yes. Thank you for asking." Your friends and family will be glad there is something concrete they can do to help you through this time, and you will have time and energy to attend to getting better.

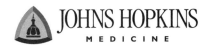

CHAPTER 7

JOHNS HOPKINS
M E D I C I N E

SURVIVING CERVICAL CANCER— RE-ENGAGING IN MIND AND BODY HEALTH AFTER TREATMENT

Your surgery is over and/or your course of radiation is completed! The move from being a patient to being a survivor can be both frightening and thrilling at the same time. When the surgery is finished and/or the radiation treatments end, a sense of panic may set in out of fear that the medical providers are no longer keeping such a close watch over you. You may start to feel hypervigilant about your body, worrying that every twinge represents a recurrence. Anytime a friend or relative is diagnosed with cancer, you will likely feel a wave of emotions as you recall how you felt when you were first diagnosed. If a friend dies from cancer, you may be gripped with worry that it will happen to you as well. Whenever a doctor's appointment is scheduled or an anniversary of the diagnosis or surgery approaches, these fears may come rushing forward.

How you manage these feelings is an individual decision. Some women find that support groups for cancer survivors are very helpful. These groups can help you realize that your feelings are normal reactions to what you have been through and can offer insight from others who have walked the same path you have. Other women prefer to rely on the support and care of their friends and family. Some women find that volunteering to help educate other women about cervical cancer prevention helps them as they become a survivor while providing a way to help others and give back some of the help they received during their treatment.

Scheduling and going to each follow-up appointment may be stressful because you are worried that the doctor will find evidence of a recurrence, and it may bring back a rush of emotions and memories from when you were first diagnosed. However, it is very important to have follow-ups with your gynecologic oncologist for the rest of your life. It is also important to note that recurrences found early are more likely to be treatable—so keep your follow-up appointments!

As you transition from being a patient to being a survivor, it would be great if all the side effects of your treatment stayed on the patient side of the equation. However, on top of the emotional adjustment you will be making, your body will also still be making adjustments over the next few months. You should not expect to feel entirely back to "normal" for several months after completing your treatment. Symptoms such as fatigue can linger for several months. In addition, some of the side effects of therapy can be permanent and your "normal" after treatment may not be the same as before treatment.

If you were premenopausal and had your ovaries removed or irradiated, you will likely experience menopause. Symptoms can include hot flashes, vaginal dryness, and irritability. While doctors used to think that all women should be on hormone replacement therapy, recent research has shown that hormone replacement therapy may increase the risk of strokes or breast cancer. However, it is a slightly different picture when the hormones are replacing hormones that your ovaries would have been making if they hadn't been removed. You should talk with your doctor about whether hormone replacement is appropriate for you.

Your sexuality may also be affected by both your cancer and the treatment of your cancer. Surgery can lead to vaginal shortening, as can radiation. Radiation may also cause your vagina to become dryer and scarred. These changes may make you more likely to have some bleeding with intercourse. And of course, anytime you see any vaginal bleeding, you are likely to worry that you have a recurrence. All this can lead to a lot of anxiety! Working with a dilator can be helpful, and frank, open discussions with your partner are also important.

Radiation can leave you with other long-term side effects as well. Bladder irritation and blood in your urine can last for a while after treatment. Bowel irritation leading to diarrhea or blood in your stools can also occur for a while. You should tell your doctors if you are having these problems so they can make sure nothing else is going on.

Doing everything you can to keep yourself healthy can be empowering as you move from being a patient to being a survivor. You have overcome one obstacle. Now is a great time to embrace a new, healthy lifestyle. Good nutrition and regular exercise are important to your overall health.

It is important to keep up with screening for other cancers too. While the thought of being diagnosed with another cancer is terrifying, remember that cancers caught early are much easier to treat. You should have a mammogram yearly if you are over 40 years old. If you are 50 years of age or older, you should have screening for colon cancer, usually by colonoscopy.

It is especially important that you stop smoking if you are a smoker. Not only does smoking increase the risk of developing cervical cancer, but it also increases the risk of it recurring! Give yourself the best chance of staying disease-free and quit smoking. It can be very difficult, and the average smoker has to make several attempts before they successfully quit. But it's worth it! Besides decreasing your risk of recurrent cervical cancer, you decrease your risk of lung and bladder cancer and the risk of emphysema. Talk to your doctor about different medications to help you quit by decreasing your cravings. Set a quit date and make sure your friends know about it. Have them remind you how important it is to your health that you quit smoking. Set aside the money that you would be spending each day on cigarettes, and after a month, several months, or a year treat yourself to something nice with that money. Figure out your triggers for smoking. Do you always smoke when you drive? When you talk on the phone? Then make sure you have something else to do with your hands during those times. For example, keep lollipops in the car, or keep a pen and paper by the phone to doodle with. Quitting smoking will significantly decrease your risk of recurrence and make you a much healthier person overall.

Surviving cancer can have some positive long-term side effects as well. After coming through this ordeal, you are seeing the world with new eyes. Coming face to face with your own mortality can make you take a step back and reassess who you are, what is important to you, and who you want to be. You may decide to make some changes in your life: go back to school, change careers, work less.

Many women who survive cancer report that their enjoyment of life eventually becomes greater than before their diagnosis because they realize how much their family and friends mean to them. They see life in a new way and savor the chance to strengthen their relationships with the people who mean the most to them. Things that once seemed like big problems now seem insignificant when compared to cancer. Life after cancer is certainly different than life before cancer, and it holds big challenges. However, it also holds possibilities for a fresh start to a brighter, more fulfilling future.

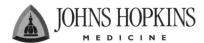

CHAPTER 8

MANAGING RISK—WHAT IF MY CANCER COMES BACK?

Concern that your cancer has recurred will stay with you for a long time. Every time you feel an extra twinge, you may worry that the cancer has returned and has now spread. Understanding the risk of recurrence, making sure to follow up regularly with your doctor, and knowing what signs to look for can help you manage these fears.

After you have finished treatment, you will enter "surveillance." This doesn't mean that someone in a trench coat will follow you around, but rather that you will have regularly scheduled appointments with your gynecologic oncologist. If you had radiation, you will likely also have follow-up appointments with your radiation oncologist. Usually, you will have an examination every 3 months for 2 years and then every 6 months for another 3 years. After 5 years, you "graduate" to yearly follow-ups. A pelvic examination and a Pap smear are usually sufficient to check for recurrences. Imaging studies (such as CAT scans) may be performed, but their usefulness is unclear.

Most women who are going to have recurrences experience them within the first 2 years after diagnosis. The risk of recurrence is higher the more advanced your cancer was at the time of diagnosis. Recurrences can be located near the initial cancer (local) or in a new location (distant).

Recurrences can present with vaginal bleeding. You should notify your doctor of this development as well as blood in your urine or bowel movements. Constant pain in your side (flank), where your kidneys are, can be a sign that recurrence has blocked the tubes that lead from your kidney to your bladder. Tell your doctor if you have flank pain that persists more than a few days. Cervical cancer can also recur in bones, which usually causes pain. If you have any pain that remains intense over several days, you should let your doctor know about it.

Treatment of recurrent cervical cancer depends on both the location of the recurrence and your prior therapies. If your recurrence is within the pelvis, your doctor will typically give a type of treatment that you have not had yet. If you had surgery in the past, radiation (with weekly chemotherapy) is usually given. If you have already had radiation to the pelvis, however, chemotherapy or surgery is usually recommended. Patients often ask why they can have surgery and chemotherapy multiple times but can only receive radiation to an area once. There is a limit to the amount of radiation the body can safely tolerate. In order to kill the cancer cells, the radiation oncologist gives enough radiation to reach that limit. Your body always "remembers" the original radiation, and if you receive additional radiation, you greatly increase your risk of significant complications. So for cervical cancer patients who have a recurrence after radiation, chemotherapy is typically recommended. Surgery may be a possibility but only in specific situations.

If a recurrence is local, relatively small, and does not extend to the pelvic bones, and if there is no other evidence of disease elsewhere, an exenteration may be an option. The surgery section in Chapter 3 offers more details about the exenteration process.

If the recurrence is blocking one of your ureters (the tubes that run from your kidney to your bladder), you may need a percutaneous nephrostomy. In this procedure, a doctor inserts a tube through the skin of your back and into your kidney. Your urine then drains into a bag.

Distant recurrences are also called metastases. Cervical cancer can spread to lymph nodes, lungs, and bones, among other places. This does not mean you have lung or bone cancer but rather that cervical cancer cells have gone to those areas. If the recurrence is only in one area, radiation to that area and/or surgery to remove it might be possible. Chemotherapy is another option. Many different chemotherapy drugs have been tried, and about 15–40% of women will see some response with chemotherapy. Treatment with two chemotherapy medications at the same time may increase the chances of a response but may also increase the side effects. Each type of chemotherapy has a different schedule and different side effects, so you need to talk with your doctor about which chemotherapy you would be receiving.

Another option for women who have recurrent disease is a clinical trial (see Chapter 3 for more about clinical trials). If you are interested in participating in a trial, you should ask your doctor if there are any available at your hospital. If not, the National Cancer Institute is an outstanding resource, or you can ask your doctor to help you find a research trial.

In general, recurrent disease is more challenging to treat than when it is first diagnosed. Early-stage cervical cancer is curable in the majority of cases. Locally advanced cervical cancer (Stage II and III) can sometimes be cured. Occasionally, cervical cancer recurrences can be cured with either radical surgery or radiation. However, the typical experience with recurrent disease is unfortunately not very good. While recurrent disease can sometimes be controlled, the vast majority of times the cancer returns or progresses at some point. Despite the very limited chance of a cure, treatment for recurrent disease is reasonable because it can lengthen your survival and improve your quality of life.

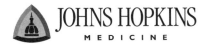

CHAPTER 9

My Cancer Isn't Curable—
What Now?

I t is devastating to hear that your cancer has spread. Learning that your cancer is not curable is terrifying and will require a shift in how you think about your treatments.

When cervical cancer has spread, the goal of treatment shifts from cure to control. As mentioned previously, the outcome for primary cervical cancer is actually very good, with cure rates of approximately 70%. However if the cancer does recur, the option for cure is usually no longer available. The exception to this rule is a local recurrence (at the top of the vagina), treated with an exenteration.

Therapy attempts to control the cancer for as long as possible while still maintaining good quality of life. It is important to have a frank talk with your doctor about what to expect. Metastatic disease can often be controlled for a period of time, but it cannot be cured. It can be difficult to hear, but having realistic expectations is important so you can make informed choices about treatment options and mentally prepare yourself for the road ahead. You shouldn't give up hope. Some women live a long time with recurrent disease—treatments can work better than expected and symptoms that are very bothersome can be treated—but you may need to shift the focus of your hope and plans.

Your physician is there to be supportive and to maximize your quality of life. Doctor visits about recurrent disease are challenging. Your physician is present to provide emotional support in what is obviously a difficult time. In addition, your doctor wants to help form an appropriate plan of action based not only on the extent of recurrent disease, but also on your view of what is the right approach. Sometimes it takes more than one visit to achieve both of these goals.

There is no right or wrong way to treat recurrent or metastatic cancer. Your choice of therapies depends on your priorities. What might be right for one patient may not be right for another. The pathway you choose is up to you, and as your treatments proceed, there are always opportunities to reassess whether that path is still right for you.

The goal of the most aggressive treatment path is to give you as much time as possible. The stress is on quantity of life. Patients pursue treatments no matter how difficult they are, even if there is only a limited possibility that they will buy them some more time. Some women, especially those with young children, may prefer this as the course of treatment. Particularly when the diagnosis of recurrent or metastatic cancer has just been made, some women want to drive as hard as possible against their cancer. It is important to remember that all treatments have side effects; aggressive chemotherapy can make you feel tired and ill, and surgery can mean you are in the hospital or recovering for a long time. There is no point in taking treatment for treatment's sake if it is just making you feel sicker. But if fighting tooth and nail against your cancer is what you need to do, then be aggressive. Just make sure you reassess as you go through therapy. Part of reassessing treatment is determining the costs and benefits. How much of your time do you need to invest? How much extra time could you receive?

At the other end of the spectrum is hospice. Hospice is a philosophy that stresses quality of life over quantity of life and aims to take care of your emotional and physical symptoms. The goal is always to make sure you are as comfortable as possible. If treatment doesn't improve the quality of your time, then you shouldn't undergo it. Patients don't receive aggressive treatments such as surgery, chemotherapy, or radiation. They do receive pain medicines, antinausea medicine, and anti-anxiety medication.

In hospice programs, nurses and doctors work to make sure that your pain is controlled, that other symptoms are taken care of, and that you and your family have the emotional support you need. Hospice services can be provided in your home or in an inpatient setting, depending on what type of services you need. Unfortunately, all too often people wait until very late before turning to hospice. Hospice doesn't mean you've "given up." Hospice is both a recognition that current available treatments will not provide much, if any, benefit and an effort to focus on getting the most quality out of the time you have left once you've decided not to continue with aggressive treatment.

Discussions about hospice can be very emotional for you and your friends and family, as well as your physician, but these conversations may be among the most important you will have with your doctor.

In order to recommend hospice, your physician needs to estimate that your life expectancy is less than 6 months. Life expectancy is an estimation. No one has a crystal ball to predict the future. Some patients are on hospice for longer than 6 months. Some patients are on hospice for less than 6 months. Even if you are not yet ready for hospice, it is often very valuable to have a discussion with hospice providers. That way you can make a more informed decision if hospice becomes a recommendation in the future. Most hospice patients and families wish that they had started hospice sooner.

Between these two paths, there is a lot of room. You may decide you do not want to be very aggressive but still want to have some treatments, as long as they do not interfere too much with your quality of life. For instance, you may decide to try some chemotherapy, working with your doctor to see which type would be relatively easy to tolerate. Assess each treatment option, and decide whether the costs outweigh the benefits.

Regardless which path you pursue, it is important to have your symptoms well controlled. Some women avoid telling their doctor about symptoms for fear that the doctor will give them bad news. But if progression of your disease is causing you pain or nausea, hiding the information from your physician will not make the symptoms any better. Sharing your symptoms allows you and your physician to plan accordingly and to get your symptoms under better control. Some women also worry that taking pain medications will lead to addiction. Although you may become tolerant of your pain medications (meaning that over time you need more medication to give you the same amount of relief), patients taking medication for cancer pain do not become addicted. It is best to take pain medications on a schedule so that you stay on top of the pain, rather than letting it sneak up on you and get out of control and then having to regain control. The same is true for antinausea medications.

Although it is difficult to consider, catastrophic events can happen, especially as one approaches the end of the disease course. If the cancer progresses, it can lead to a situation where your heart stops beating or you stop breathing. Advance directives or a living will are legal documents that allow you to convey your decisions about end-of-life care ahead of time. It is important to think about whether you would want to be resuscitated or not in these situations. Many times, patients and doctors are afraid to have this discussion and wait until it is late in the course of treatment, but it is a good idea to think through what you would want and make sure that your family and your doctors understand your wishes. In the United States, if individuals stop breathing or if their hearts stop beating, we assume they would want "everything" done to save their lives. Thus we perform CPR, including electric shocks to try to restart their hearts, and intubation, which involves inserting a breathing tube into their throats. While these methods almost always work on TV, in real life, especially when people are already sick, they work much less often. And if they do "work," the patient can end up on a ventilator (breathing machine) or in the intensive care unit for a long time. Remember, you always have the option to decline CPR, and, in fact, declining life-saving methods often is a completely appropriate choice. If you do not want

CPR, let your doctors and family know so your wishes can be respected. The advanced directive is the formal legal document to explain your desires for end-of-life care. However, you can also have a conversation with your physician to explain these details. A conversation sometimes allows for a fuller discussion of all the possibilities. A written advanced directive ensures there is documentation of your desires, especially if you cannot communicate with your healthcare providers. You can also designate a healthcare proxy to make decisions for you if you are unable to do so. If you do not designate a healthcare proxy, the hospital will sometimes need to assign one. Unless you specify otherwise, your family has priority over your friends, and certain relatives have priority over others. Ideally, it is best to communicate your end-of-life preferences to your healthcare team, both verbally and in writing.

Talking with friends and family can be difficult. Often they are not as prepared for the news as you are. After all, this is your cancer journey, and you have been emotionally dealing with it since your diagnosis. Talking with young children can be especially difficult. Children are very perceptive, however, and lying to them will only breed distrust and fear. Often the hospital has a social worker who may be able to help you plan for this conversation. Other good resources are survivor support groups or your minister, if you have one. If you decide to pursue hospice care, they often can provide support and advice for family members.

Being diagnosed with recurrent or metastatic cervical cancer also will lead to a lot of emotional turmoil for you. It is difficult and painful to face your own mortality and to evaluate what you have accomplished in life, or what you have left undone. It is a time to reflect and come to peace with your life. Many people find it therapeutic to reach out to loved ones and make sure they know how much they mean to you and to extend a hand of forgiveness to those with whom you have parted ways. If you are a religious person, your minister may be able to help. The hospital social worker, support groups, and loved ones are also important sources of strength for this process.

Being diagnosed with recurrent or metastatic cancer can be seen as a rare, albeit very difficult, opportunity. We will all die, and sudden accidents can happen. In contrast, you have the opportunity to reflect, to come to a sense of peace, and to settle affairs with your friends and family.

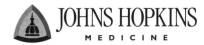

CHAPTER 10

CERVICAL CANCER
IN OLDER ADULTS

GARY R. SHAPIRO, MD

The average age of women with cancer of the cervix is around 50 years. However, one in five women with cervical cancer is at least 75 years of age. Although the wide use of the Pap smear has dramatically decreased the frequency of cervical cancer in developed countries such as the United States, the older population remains at risk.

Older adults with cancer often have other chronic health problems and may be taking multiple medications that can affect their cancer treatment plan. Prejudice, misunderstanding, and limited access to clinical trials often prevent older patients from getting the timely cancer treatment they need. Older women may not have adequate screening for cervical cancer, and when a cancer is found, it is too often ignored or undertreated. As a result, older women often have more advanced cancer and worse outcomes than younger patients.

WHY IS THERE MORE CANCER IN OLDER PEOPLE?

The organs in our body are made up of cells. Cells divide and multiply as the body needs them. Cancer develops when cells in a part of the body grow out of control. The body has a number of ways of repairing damaged control mechanisms, but as we age, these methods do not work as well. Although our healthier lifestyles have allowed us to avoid death from infection, heart attack, and stroke, we may now live long enough for a cancer to develop. People who live longer have increased exposure to cancer-causing agents (carcinogens) in the environment. Aging decreases the body's ability to protect us from these carcinogens and to repair cells that are damaged by these and other processes.

CERVICAL CANCER IS DIFFERENT IN OLDER WOMEN

The biology of cervical cancer is different in older women than in younger women. As women age, there is an increased risk of in situ cervical cancer progressing to invasive cancer; there is also a lower rate of regression of cervical precancer. While older women are less likely to have active HPV infection than younger women, older women do appear to be at risk for a reactivation of a HPV infection from their younger years.

DECISION MAKING: 7 PRACTICAL STEPS

1. GET A DIAGNOSIS

No matter how "typical" the signs and symptoms, first impressions are sometimes wrong. That unusual vaginal bleeding or pelvic pain that you are having may well be benign. A diagnosis helps you and your family understand what to expect and how to prepare for the future, even if you cannot get curative treatment. Knowing the diagnosis also helps your doctor treat your symptoms better. Many people find "not knowing" very hard and are relieved when they finally have an explanation for their symptoms. Sometimes a frail patient is obviously dying, and diagnostic studies can be an additional burden. In such cases, it may be quite reasonable to focus on symptom relief (palliation) without knowing the details of the diagnosis.

2. KNOW THE CANCER'S STAGE

The cancer's stage defines your prognosis and treatment options. No one can make informed decisions without knowing the stage. Just as there may be times when the burdens of diagnostic studies may be too great, it may also be appropriate to do without full staging in very frail, dying patients.

Cervical cancer is staged clinically, not surgically. As it is in younger patients, stage is determined based on evidence of the cancer spreading outside the cervix through an exam, chest X-ray, or kidney scan. Factors, such as the depth of the tumor, the presence or absence of cancer in lymph nodes, or spread (metastasis) to other organs not seen on a chest X-ray are important in determining prognosis, but do not affect the cancer's stage. However, in order to predict the impact of cervical cancer on your life expectancy and quality of life, doctors take into account both the cancer's stage and other evidence of spread outside the cervix, even if it does not alter the stage.

3. KNOW YOUR LIFE EXPECTANCY

Anticancer treatment should be considered if you are likely to live long enough to experience symptoms or premature death from cervical cancer. If your life expectancy is so short that the cancer will not significantly affect it, there may be no reason to treat your cancer.

However, chronological age (how old you are) should not be the only determinant of how your cancer should, or should not, be treated. Despite advanced age, women who are relatively healthy often have a life expectancy that is longer than their life expectancy with cervical cancer. The average 70-year-old woman is likely to live another 16 years. A similar 85-year-old can expect to live an additional 6 years and remain independent most of that time. Even an unhealthy 75-year-old woman probably will live 5 more years, which is long enough to suffer symptoms and early death from metastatic cervical cancer.

4. UNDERSTAND THE GOALS

The Goals of Treatment

It is important to be clear whether the goal of treatment is cure (surgery or radiation therapy, possibly with chemotherapy, for early stage cervical cancer) or palliation (treatment for incurable advanced cervical cancer). If the goal is palliation, you need to understand if the treatment plan will extend your life, control your symptoms, or both. How likely is it to achieve these goals, and how long will you enjoy its benefits?

When the goal of treatment is palliation, chemotherapy should never be administered without defined endpoints and timelines. It should be clear to everyone what "counts" as success, how it will be determined (for example, a symptom controlled or a smaller mass on your CAT scan), and when. You and your family should understand what your options are at each step and how likely each option is to meet your goals. If treatment goals are not clear, ask your doctor to explain them in words you understand.

The Goals of the Patient

In addition to the traditional goals of tumor response, increased survival, and symptom control, older cancer patients often have goals related to quality of life. These goals may include physical and intellectual independence, spending quality time with family, taking trips, staying out of the hospital, or even economic stability. At times, palliative care or hospice may meet these goals better than active anticancer treatment. In addition to the medical team, older patients often turn to family, friends, and clergy to help guide them.

5. DETERMINE IF YOU ARE FIT OR FRAIL

Deciding how to treat cervical cancer in someone who is older requires a thorough understanding of her general health and social situation. Decisions about cancer treatment should never focus on age alone.

Age Is Not a Number

Your actual age (chronological age) has limited influence on how cancer will respond to therapy or its prognosis. Biological changes and other changes associated with aging are more reliable in estimating an individual's vigor and life expectancy as well as the risk of treatment complications. These changes include malnutrition, loss of muscle mass and strength, depression, dementia, falls, social isolation, and the ability to accomplish daily activities such as dressing, bathing, eating, shopping, housekeeping, and managing one's finances or medication.

Chronic Illnesses

Older cancer patients are likely to have chronic illnesses (comorbidities) that affect their life expectancy; the more they have, the greater the effect. This effect has very little impact on the behavior of the cancer itself, but studies do show that comorbidity has a major impact on treatment outcome and its side effects.

6. BALANCE BENEFIT AND HARM

Fit older cervical cancer patients respond to treatment similarly to their younger counterparts. However, a word of caution is in order. Until recently, few studies included older individuals, and it may not be appropriate to apply these findings to the diverse group of older cancer patients.

The side effects of cancer treatment are never less in the elderly. In addition to the standard side effects, there are significant age-related toxicities to consider. Though most of these are more a function of frailty than chronological age, even the fittest senior cannot avoid the physical effects of aging. In addition to the changes in fat and muscle you see in the mirror, there are age-related changes in your kidney, liver, and digestive (gastrointestinal) function. These changes affect how your body absorbs and metabolizes anticancer drugs and other medicines. The average older woman takes many different medicines (to control, for example, high blood pressure, high cholesterol, osteoporosis, diabetes, arthritis, etc.). This "polypharmacy" can cause undesirable side effects as the many drugs interact with each other and the anticancer medications.

7. GET INVOLVED

Healthcare providers and family members often under-estimate the physical and mental abilities of older people and their willingness to face chronic and life-threatening conditions. Studies clearly show that older patients want detailed and easily understood information about potential treatments and alternatives. Patients and families may consider cancer untreatable in the aged and may not understand the possibilities offered by treatment.

While patients with dementia pose a unique challenge, they are frequently capable of participating in goal setting and simple discussions about treatment side effects and logistics. Caring family members and friends are often able to share the patient's life story so that healthcare workers can work with them to make decisions consistent with the patient's values and desires. This of course is no substitute for a well thought out and properly executed living will or healthcare proxy.

While it is hard to face the possibility of life-threatening events at any age, it is always better to be prepared and to "put your affairs in order." In addition to estate planning and wills, it is critical that you outline your wishes regarding medical care at the end of life and make legal provisions for someone to make those decisions if you are unable to make them for yourself.

TREATING CERVICAL CANCER

YOU NEED A TEAM

Cancer care changes rapidly, and it is hard for the generalist to keep up to date, so referral to a specialist is essential. The needs of an older cancer patient often extend beyond the doctor's office and the traditional services provided by visiting nurses. These needs may include transportation, nutrition, emotional, financial, physical, or spiritual support. When an older woman with cervical cancer is the primary caregiver for a frail or ill spouse, grandchildren, or other family members, special attention is necessary to provide for their needs as well. Older cancer patients cared for in geriatric oncology programs benefit from multi-disciplinary teams of oncologists, geriatricians, psychiatrists, pharmacists, physiatrists, social workers, nurses, clergy, and dietitians, all working together as a team to identify and manage the stressors that can limit effective cancer treatment.

SURGERY

Surgery (hysterectomy or cold knife cone) for cervical cancer is a relatively low-risk operation and the standard of care for all women with very early stage cervical cancer, regardless of age. When cervical cancer is more advanced but still confined to the cervix, surgery and radiation are equally effective and the "right decision" depends on many factors. You and your physician need to discuss the advantages and disadvantages of both approaches. Like other treatment options, surgery in some older women may involve risks related to decreases in body organ function (especially in the heart and lungs), and it is essential that the surgeon and anesthetist work closely with the primary care physician (or a consultant) to fully assess and treat these problems before, during, and after the operation. Because future childbearing is not an issue for older women, most cervical cancer operations (see Chapter 3) will involve removing the cervix and uterus (hysterectomy).

RADIATION THERAPY

Radiation therapy may be an effective option for some women who have early stage cervical cancers, especially if the patient cannot tolerate surgery. It is also used as an adjunct to surgery (often with chemotherapy) in women who, despite having early stage disease, are at high risk for recurrence (see Chapter 3). Radiation (often with chemotherapy) is also the treatment of choice for most advanced cervical cancers. In addition, radiation therapy is particularly useful in treating recurrent cervical cancer patients who have not received radiation in the past. Healthy older women usually tolerate radiation therapy quite well, and even frail patients may find the side effects acceptable.

Though studies in older women have found no significant increase in the side effects from radiation therapy, the fatigue that often accompanies radiation therapy can be quite profound in the elderly, even in those who are fit. Often the logistic details (like daily travel to the hospital for a 6-week course of treatment) are the hardest for older people. It is important that you discuss these potential problems with your family and social worker prior to starting radiation therapy.

Although radiation therapy may sound more appealing than an operation, surgery is actually quicker and usually has fewer long-term side effects. Radiation therapy may contribute to urinary problems or difficulties with bowel movements and can sometimes make sex difficult or painful by causing scarring or shortening of the vagina. It may be hard for you to discuss these issues with your doctor, but be sure that you do. Many people make the mistake of assuming that sex is not important to older women.

CHEMOTHERAPY

Chemotherapy is usually used as a sensitizer (chemosensitization) with radiation therapy in women with more advanced cervical cancer that has not yet metastasized. Chemotherapy can also be given by itself to treat metastatic (stage IV) cervical cancer or certain types of recurrent cervical cancer.

Older cancer patients who are not frail respond to chemotherapy similarly to their younger counterparts. Though the side effects of cancer treatment are never less burdensome in the elderly, they can be managed by oncologists, especially geriatric oncologists, who work in teams with others who specialize in the care of the elderly. With appropriate care, healthy older women do just as well with chemotherapy as younger women.

Advances in supportive care (antinausea medicines and blood cell growth factors) have significantly decreased the side effects of chemotherapy and have improved the safety and the quality of life of older women with cervical cancer. Nonetheless, there is risk, especially in frail patients.

Platinol AQ is usually used when chemotherapy is given with radiation therapy. It serves to sensitize the tumor to the effects of the radiation (see Chapter 3), but this benefit is not without its downsides. Platinol AQ can cause severe side effects in older patients, especially fatigue and problems related to the kidney (nephrotoxicity). Those treated with Platinol AQ chemotherapy require large amounts of intravenous fluid hydration, which can cause congestive heart failure in people with heart problems.

Alone or in combination, Platinol AQ, Paraplatin, Taxol, Hycamtin (topotecan), and Garamycin (gentamicin) are the most commonly used agents for metastatic cervical cancer. Healthy older patients can receive the same regimens as their younger counterparts, including those that are cisplatin-based. Taxol and Paraplatin are often the first regimen chosen for metastatic disease and this combination is usually well tolerated. Older women whose cervical cancers have progressed despite first-line therapy have the same benefit from chemotherapy as their younger counterparts. They should not be excluded from receiving chemotherapy for advanced cervical cancer. Preference should be given to chemotherapeutic drugs with safer profiles, such as weekly taxane regimens and Paraplatin. Single-agent therapy is less toxic and may be a reasonable palliative alternative to combination chemotherapy in some elderly patients.

COMMON TREATMENT COMPLICATIONS IN THE ELDERLY

Anemia (low red blood cell count) is common in the elderly, especially the frail elderly. It decreases the effectiveness of chemotherapy and often causes fatigue, falls, cognitive decline (for example, dementia, disorientation, or confusion), and heart problems. Therefore, it is essential that anemia be recognized and corrected with red blood cell transfusions or the appropriate use of erythropoiesis-stimulating agents like Procrit and Epogen (epoetin) or Aranesp.

Myelosuppression (low white blood cell count) is also common in older patients receiving chemotherapy or radiation. Older patients with myelosuppression develop life-threatening infections more often than younger patients, and they may need to be treated in the hospital for many days. The liberal use of granulopoietic growth factors (or

G-CSF, including Neupogen [filgrastim] and Neulasta) decreases the risk of infection and makes it possible for older women to receive full doses of potentially curative adjuvant chemotherapy.

Mucositis (mouth sores) and diarrhea can cause severe dehydration in older patients who often are already dehydrated due to inadequate fluid intake and diuretics ("water pills" for high blood pressure or heart failure). Careful monitoring, the liberal use of antidiarrheal agents (Imodium), and oral and intravenous fluids are essential components of the management of older cancer patients.

Kidney function declines as we age. Some of the medicines that older patients take to treat both their cancer (for example, Platinol AQ, Paraplatin, Zometa [zoledronic acid], NSAIDs) and noncancer-related problems might further worsen kidney function. The dehydration that often accompanies cancer and its treatment can put additional stress on the kidneys. Fortunately, it is often possible to minimize these effects by carefully selecting and dosing appropriate drugs, managing polypharmacy, and preventing dehydration.

Neurotoxicity and cognitive effects (chemo-brain) can be profoundly debilitating in patients who are already cognitively impaired (demented, disoriented, confused, etc.). Elderly patients with a history of falling, hearing loss, or peripheral neuropathy (nerve damage from, for example, diabetes) have decreased energy and are highly vulnerable to neurotoxic chemotherapy like the taxanes or platinum compounds. Many of the medicines used to control nausea (antiemetics) or decrease the side effects of certain chemotherapeutic agents are also potential neurotoxins. These medicines include dexamethasone (psychosis and agitation), ranitidine (agitation), diphenhydramine, and some of the antiemetics (sedation).

Fatigue is a near universal complaint of older cancer patients. It is particularly a problem for those who are socially isolated or dependent upon others for help with activities of daily living. It is not necessarily related to depression, but can be. Depression is quite common in the elderly. In contrast to younger patients who often respond to a cancer diagnosis with anxiety, depression is the more common disorder in older cancer patients. With proper support and medical attention, many of these patients can safely receive anticancer treatment.

Heart problems increase with age, and it is no surprise that older cancer patients have an increased risk of cardiac complications from intensive surgery, radiation, and chemotherapy. Patients treated with Platinol AQ chemotherapy require large amounts of intravenous fluid hydration, which can cause congestive heart failure in patients with heart problems; they need careful monitoring.

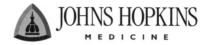

CHAPTER 11

JOHNS HOPKINS
M E D I C I N E

TRUSTED RESOURCES— FINDING ADDITIONAL INFORMATION ABOUT CERVICAL CANCER AND ITS TREATMENT

National Cancer Institute
1-800-4-CANCER
http://www.cancer.gov

This organization provides information about all types of cancer, including excellent information about cervical cancer, what it is, how it is treated, and where various treatment options are provided. You can request free information by calling the toll-free number.

Specific information for patients and family members seeking to learn more about cervical cancer, treatment options, and current clinical trials can be found at http://www.cancer.gov/cancertopics/types/cervical.

American Cancer Society

1-800-ACS-2345

http://www.cancer.org/docroot/CRI/CRI_2_3x. asp?dt=8

National Cervical Cancer Coalition

http://www.nccc-online.org

This Web site provides information, with an emphasis on personal outreach support, for women and their families dealing with cervical cancer.

Women's Cancer Network

http://www.wcn.org/

This organization provides women information on research, risks, prevention, and treatment for gynecologic cancers, and empowers them to make informed decisions regarding their health care.

Fertile Hope

http://www.fertilehope.org

Fertile Hope is an organization dedicated to providing reproductive information, support, and hope to cancer patients and survivors whose medical treatments present the risk of infertility.

WHERE CAN I GET HELP WITH FINANCIAL OR LEGAL CONCERNS?

Accompanying any serious illness are questions and concerns related to expenses incurred as a result of treatment, health insurance questions that can be overwhelming to try to understand or resolve alone, and sometimes even legal questions related to employment or financial matters. The following is a list of national resources to aid you in addressing these types of concerns.

Cancer*Care*

> http://1-212-712-8400
> 1-800-813-HOPE
> Email: info@cancercare.org
> http://www.cancercare.org

Cancer*Care* is a national nonprofit organization that provides free, professional assistance to people with any type of cancer and to their families. This organization offers education, one-on-one counseling, financial assistance for nonmedical expenses, and referrals to community services.

National Coalition for Cancer Survivorship (NCCS)

> 1-301-650-8868
> 1-877-NCSS-YES
> Email: info@canceradvocacy.org
> http://www.canceradvocacy.org

This network of independent groups and individuals provides information and resources about cancer support, advocacy, and quality-of-life issues as well as helps cancer patients deal with insurance or job discrimination and other related legal matters.

Patient Advocate Foundation (PAF)

> 1-757-873-6668
> 1-800-532-5274
> Email: patient@pinn.net
> http://www.patientadvocate.org

This organization provides educational information about managed care/insurance issues and legal counseling on debt intervention, job discrimination issues, and insurance denials of coverage.

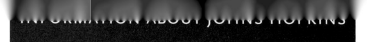

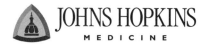

INFORMATION ABOUT JOHNS HOPKINS

The Kelly Gynecologic Oncology Service at Johns Hopkins
Appointment line: (410) 502-4245
Kelly Gynecologic Oncology Service email:
kgos@jhmi.edu

The Kelly Gynecologic Oncology Service offers comprehensive, state-of-the-art cervical cancer diagnosis and treatment.

About Johns Hopkins Medicine
Johns Hopkins Medicine unites physicians and scientists of the Johns Hopkins University School of Medicine with the organizations, health professionals, and facilities of the Johns Hopkins Health System. Its mission is to improve

the health of the community and the world by setting the standard of excellence in medical education, research, and clinical care. Diverse and inclusive, Johns Hopkins Medicine has provided international leadership in the education of physicians and medical scientists in biomedical research and in the application of medical knowledge to sustain health since The Johns Hopkins Hospital opened in 1889.

If you plan to be evaluated or treated at Johns Hopkins, you will probably meet Dr. Giuntoli. He interacts with patients on a daily basis through evaluation, treatment planning, and management of gynecologic cancers.

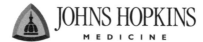

FURTHER READING

100 Questions and Answers About Cervical Cancer, Don S. Dizon, Michael L. Krychman, and Paul A. DiSilvestro, Jones and Bartlett Publishers, 2009

GLOSSARY

Advance directives: Also called a *living will*. These are legal documents that allow you to convey your decisions about end-of-life care ahead of time.

Anemia: Low red blood cell count.

Bladder: Organ responsible for storing urine. It is located in front of the uterus and cervix.

Blood vessels: Arteries and veins. Arteries carry blood from the heart to the body. Veins carry blood back to the heart. The aorta is the main artery that carries blood directly from the heart. The abdominal aorta is the portion of the aorta that is located in the abdomen. The aorta splits in the upper pelvis and supplies blood to the pelvis and to the legs. Sometimes, physicians refer to the pelvic vessels, which include the iliac and obturator vessels. The inferior vena cava is a large vein located in the abdomen that brings blood back to the heart.

Cerclage: Procedure in which the cervix or lower part of the uterus is sewn shut with a stitch.

Cervical incompetence: Condition in which the cervix dilates too early in a pregnancy, potentially leading to preterm delivery or pregnancy loss. It is sometimes treated with a cerclage.

Cervical stenosis: Condition in which scarring causes the cervix to narrow or close. It can sometime prevent the cervix from dilating during delivery and can result in a cesarean section. It also can make it difficult to evaluate the cervix after treatment.

Cervix: The opening to the uterus. The cervix dilates when you go into labor. Both dysplasias (precancers) and cancers can be diagnosed in the cervix. Pap smears are able to detect these changes early and have dramatically decreased the number of cervical cancers diagnosed in the United States. The cervix can be removed either by itself (trachelectomy) or with the rest of the uterus (hysterectomy).

Chemosensitization: Use of a small dose of chemotherapy, usually given weekly, to make radiation therapy more successful.

Chemotherapy: Use of medication, usually placed in the vein, to treat cancer.

Cold knife cone: Cone-shaped biopsy of the cervix with a scalpel. This is usually performed for diagnosis of cervical cancer, but can be curative for dysplasias and very early (microinvasive) cancers.

Colposcopy: Procedure in which your physician takes a very close look at your cervix with a microscope (called a colposcope). Biopsies are usually done to make a diagnosis and determine treatment.

Cystoscopy: Procedure in which your physician looks in your bladder to make sure that there is no evidence of cancer in that location and also to make sure that the ureters (tubes from the kidneys to the bladder) are working well.

da Vinci Surgical System: Medical instrument that augments a surgeon's ability to perform laparoscopic surgery. The da Vinci robot gives the surgeon better optics (view of the surgical target) and better dexterity with the surgical instruments.

Dehydration: Condition where your body doesn't have enough water and salts for normal function.

Depression: A change in mood characterized by persistent sadness, inability to concentrate, insomnia, loss of appetite, feelings of helplessness and hopelessness, and even thoughts of death.

Diarrhea: Frequent, watery bowel movements.

Do not resuscitate (DNR): A request by the patient that medical staff do not perform cardiopulmonary resuscitation (CPR).

Dysplasia: A precancerous change in abnormal cells present in the lining of the cervix. These abnormal cells are identified by Pap smears. Dysplasia is caused by human papilloma virus.

Ectocervix: The outside portion of the cervix, which is lined with squamous cells.

Endocervix: The inside portion of the cervix, which is lined with glandular cells. This forms the tunnel that leads to the inside of the uterus.

Exam under anesthesia: A thorough pelvic exam that your doctor performs while you are asleep in the operating room. Because you are more comfortable than you would be in the office, your physician is better able to determine the exact extent of your disease.

Exenteration: Radical surgery performed on a small group of patients with recurrent cervical cancer. It involves removal of the bladder and rectum and can be curative in some patients. Removal of the bladder and/or rectum requires an ostomy.

Fallopian tubes: Reproductive organs that allow sperm to travel to the ovary, where an egg may be present, and allow a fertilized egg to travel to the uterus. A salpingectomy is the name of the surgery to remove the tubes.

Fatigue: Loss of normal strength and energy.

Fistula: An abnormal passageway between two organs in the body or between an organ and the exterior of the body. This can be caused by radiation, surgery, or by cancer itself.

Gynecologic oncology: Division of obstetrics and gynecology. Physicians in this area specialize in the treatment of women with cancers of the reproductive tract.

Healthcare proxy: A friend or relative who is designated by you to make healthcare decisions for you if you are unable to do so.

Human papillomavirus (HPV): A virus that causes warts, cervical dysplasia, and cancer. A vaccine is currently available to prevent HPV infection.

Hysterectomy: Surgery that removes the uterus. A total hysterectomy means removal of the uterus and the cervix. A supracervical hysterectomy refers to the removal of the uterus, but not the cervix. This is not usually performed when the patient has cervical cancer or dysplasia. A radical hysterectomy involves removal of not only the uterus and cervix, but also the ligaments that hold the cervix in place. Hysterectomies can be performed through an abdominal incision (abdominal hysterectomy), through the vagina (vaginal hysterectomy), or with laparoscopy (laparoscopic hysterectomy or laparoscopically-assisted hysterectomy). The type of hysterectomy does not refer to the removal of the tubes or ovaries.

In vitro fertilization (IVF): Also known as a "test tube" pregnancy. IVF is a process by which a woman is stimulated to produce many eggs. These eggs are harvested and then fertilized with sperm from her partner or a donor. The embryos are placed in the uterus of the patient or a surrogate, and if successful, will lead to the delivery of a full-term infant.

Kidneys: Organs responsible for making urine. You have two of them, a right and a left. They are located in the mid-abdomen, towards the back.

Laparoscopy: Also known as minimally invasive surgery. Your physician performs the surgery with use of a camera and narrow instruments, which are all inserted into the abdomen through small incisions.

Loop electrosurgical excisional procedure (LEEP): A biopsy of the cervix with a charged wire. This probably results in less damage to the cervix than a cold knife cone, but pathology results are more difficult to interpret.

Lymphadenectomy: A procedure that is used to remove lymph nodes from around vessels in the body. Lymph nodes help filter fluid as it returns from the body back to the heart. Cancer cells can get trapped in the lymph nodes. Lymphadenectomy is often performed as part of cancer surgery in order to stage the cancer (determine how far it has spread).

Lymphedema: Swelling in the arms or legs that can occur after a lymphadenectomy.

Mucositis: Mouth sores.

Myelosuppression: Inhibition of the bone marrow by chemotherapy. Bone marrow produces white blood cells, red blood cells, and platelets, so all of these factors can become depressed.

Neutropenia: Low white blood cell count.

Oophoropexy: Surgery that places the ovaries outside of the pelvis in order to avoid damage by pelvic radiation. Oophoropexy is typically performed in patients who require pelvic radiation but want to maintain ovarian function.

Ostomy: An opening or hole in the abdomen created to allow for the exit of bowel movement or urine. This is needed for a procedure called exenteration, which requires the removal of the rectum and the bladder. Ostomy bags (appliances) are usually required to collect the bowel movement or urine.

Ovaries: Also called "gonads." These are reproductive organs responsible for making eggs every month while you are having periods. You have two, a right and a left. The ovaries also make hormones, primarily estrogen and progesterone. When you go through menopause, the ovaries stop making not only eggs, but also hormones. The loss of hormones results in the symptoms of menopause such as hot flashes. Oophorectomy is the name for the surgery to remove the ovaries.

Papanicolaou (Pap) smear: Also called "cervical cytology." This test is performed as part of a woman's annual exam. It looks for abnormal cells, which may indicate the presence of cervical dysplasia or cancer. Typically the next step in the work up is a colposcopy. Pap smears have resulted in a dramatic decrease in the number of cervical cancers seen in the United States.

Parametrium: The tissue or ligaments that hold the cervix in place. This tissue is removed as part of a radical hysterectomy.

Percutaneous nephrostomy: A tube placed through the skin of the back into the kidney. The tube is placed when there is an obstruction of the ureter.

Radiation: The use of high-energy rays to treat cancer. The radiation can either be pointed at the body from the outside (external beam radiation) or can be placed in the body (brachytherapy).

Radiation cystitis: Inflammation of the bladder caused by radiation therapy.

Rectum: The distal portion of the large bowel (colon). This portion of colon stores bowel movement and is located behind the uterus and cervix.

Reproductive endocrinology and infertility: A division of obstetrics and gynecology. Physicians in this specialty treat many diseases related to hormonal imbalances of the reproductive organs. These doctors often specialize in the treatment of couples with difficulty in conceiving and carrying pregnancies to term.

Salpingo-oophorectomy: Surgery that removes the fallopian tube and ovary. Unitlateral means removal of either the right or left tube and ovary. Bilateral means that both tubes and ovaries are removed. If a patient is premenopausal and both ovaries are removed, she will go into surgical menopause (immediate). Hormone replacement may be an option. As long as one of the ovaries remains in place, the surgery itself will not cause the symptoms of menopause.

Sigmoidoscopy: Procedure in which your physician looks into your rectum and sigmoid colon to make sure that there is no evidence of disease in that location.

Surrogate: A woman willing to carry a pregnancy for another woman who is unable to carry a pregnancy.

Thrombocytopenia: A low platelet count.

Trachelectomy: A surgery that removes the cervix but does not remove the uterus. This surgery preserves fertility, so a patient can carry a pregnancy after treatment. A cerclage is placed at the time of surgery. If a patient does get pregnant after a trachelectomy, a cesarean section is required for delivery.

Ureters: Tubes that connect the kidneys to the bladder. You have two of them, a right and a left. The ends of the ureters near the bladder are very close to the cervix and because of this, they can be injured during treatment for cervical cancer.

Uterus: Often referred to as the "womb." This reproductive organ is located in the center of the pelvis and is where your baby grows when you are pregnant. Hysterectomy is the name of the surgery to remove this organ.

Vaccine: Injection that leads to immunity against an infection.

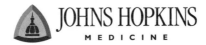

INDEX